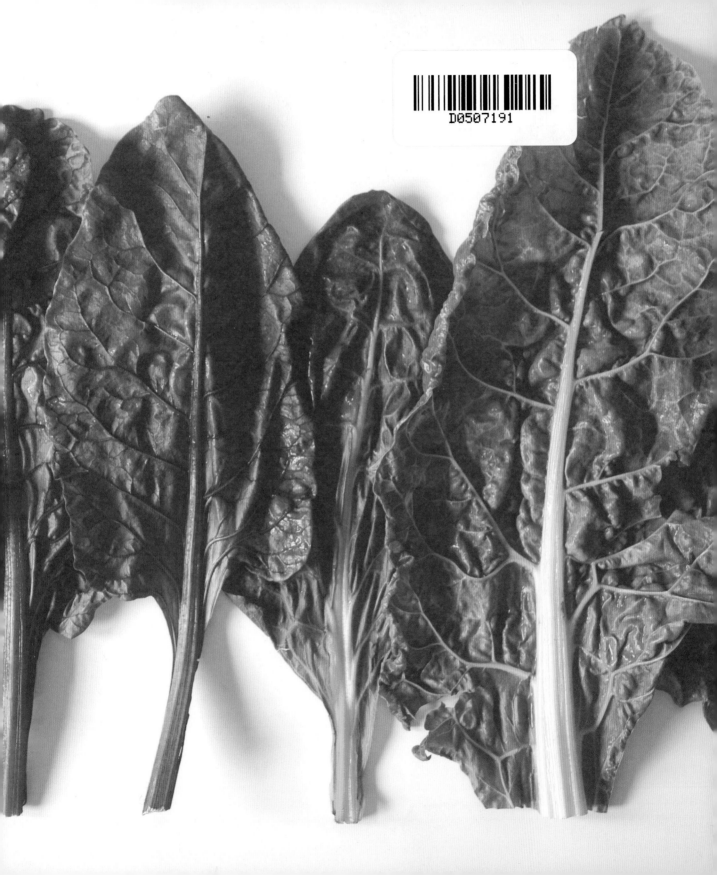

Clean Eating

More than 100 delicious whole food recipes

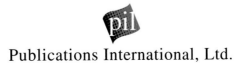

Publications International, Ltd.

Photography on pages 54, 86, 106, 136, 166 and back cover by PIL Photo Studio North.

Photographs on pages 6 and 32 © Shutterstock.com.

Pictured on the front cover *(clockwise from top left):* Heirloom Tomato Quinoa Salad *(page 56),* Beef and Pepper Kabobs *(page 108),* Zucchini Ribbon Salad *(page 156)* and Tuna Steaks with Pineapple Salsa *(page 126).*

ISBN: 978-1-68022-193-0

Library of Congress Control Number: 2015947635

Manufactured in China.

8 7 6 5 4 3 2 1

Contents

Introduction

Clean eating is not a "diet" in the typical sense; that is, it's not a crash diet. You don't have to eliminate a food group, count calories, eat like a caveman or avoid fat. The principles of clean eating are quite simple—eat foods in their natural state (or as close as possible) and avoid processed foods, refined sugars (white sugar), refined grains (white flour) and high-sodium foods—but it does take planning and commitment to implement them in your life.

Start by going through your pantry and getting rid of anything that's old or processed: half boxes of stale cereal, high-sodium soups, packaged cookies, and that one sleeve of crackers left over from your holiday party.

Plan your meals, make a list and then go grocery shopping with fresh eyes and plenty of time to read labels and explore. Pay particular attention to the produce section of your grocery store; you may be surprised to find things you've never seen before.

Keep in mind that not everything from a jar or can is bad. Look at the ingredients for many jarred salsas and you'll find that they're simply tomatoes, vegetables and seasonings. Jarred fruit packed in water, like peach slices, pineapple chunks and grapefruit sections, make it easy to snack on fruit when fresh versions are not available or you don't have time to prepare it. Organic canned beans, tomatoes and vegetables are readily available and make meal preparations much easier.

When shopping for snacks, pick apples, oranges and organic yogurt instead of chips, crackers and cookies. When you have time, make batches of Fruit Salad with Creamy Banana Dressing (page 170), Hot and Spicy Hummus (page 161) or Spicy Roasted Chickpeas (page 150) and pack them into small jars for snacking throughout the week.

TIPS FOR CLEAN EATING

Eat small meals throughout the day to keep your blood sugar and energy levels steady. If you're not going to be at home or work, pack a cooler bag with a snack. Smoothies and juices make great pick-me-ups on the run; make them in the morning and transport them in a jar or travel cup.

Use clean eating as a opportunity to make other positive lifestyle changes: start (or continue) exercising, drink lots of water and get plenty of sleep.

Be realistic. It's easy to be overwhelmed by too many rules and criteria when beginning a new eating plan, so start small and make gradual changes. When you run out of regular pasta and white rice, buy whole wheat pasta and brown rice next time. Choose oats, granola and dried fruit instead of breakfast cereal. If you take sugar in your coffee or tea, gradually reduce the amount you use until you don't need it anymore.

Use common sense when shopping. If a product has a lot of ingredients, any of them sugar and most of them unpronounceable, skip it.

When shopping for fruits, vegetables, meats and dairy, choose organic or the best quality that you can afford. Try farmers' markets for eggs and cheese, and look for produce marked "local" at the grocery store for just-picked freshness.

Quick Reference Guide
to Grocery Shopping

STOCK UP

VEGETABLES, ALL KINDS

fresh

frozen

canned

FRUIT, ALL KINDS

fresh

frozen

canned or jarred

dried

WHOLE GRAINS

barley

oats

quinoa

rice (brown)

whole grain pasta

PROTEIN

beans

beef

chicken

eggs

fish and shellfish

lamb

pork

tofu

turkey

DAIRY

butter

dairy-free milk alternatives
(soymilk, coconut milk, almond
milk, rice milk)

milk

yogurt (plain)

NUTS AND OILS

avocado oil

coconut oil

nuts (all kinds)

nut butters

olive oil

seeds (chia, flax, pumpkin,
sesame, sunflower)

SEASONINGS AND SAUCES

herbs (fresh and dried)

hot sauce

mustard

sea salt and black pepper

spices

vinegar

SWEETENERS

agave nectar

honey

maple syrup

PANTRY STAPLES

broth

canned beans

canned tomatoes and tomato
sauce

coconut milk

salsa

AVOID

PROCESSED FOODS

canned soups

chips and pretzels

fat-free dairy products

frozen pizza and meals

hot dogs

margarine

packaged shredded cheese

salad dressings

REFINED GRAINS

crackers

packaged breads

regular pasta

white rice

SUGAR

artificial sugar substitute

candy

cookies

ice cream

jams and jellies

sweetened peanut butter

soda, energy drinks and other
sugary beverages

sugary cereals

yogurt with added sugar

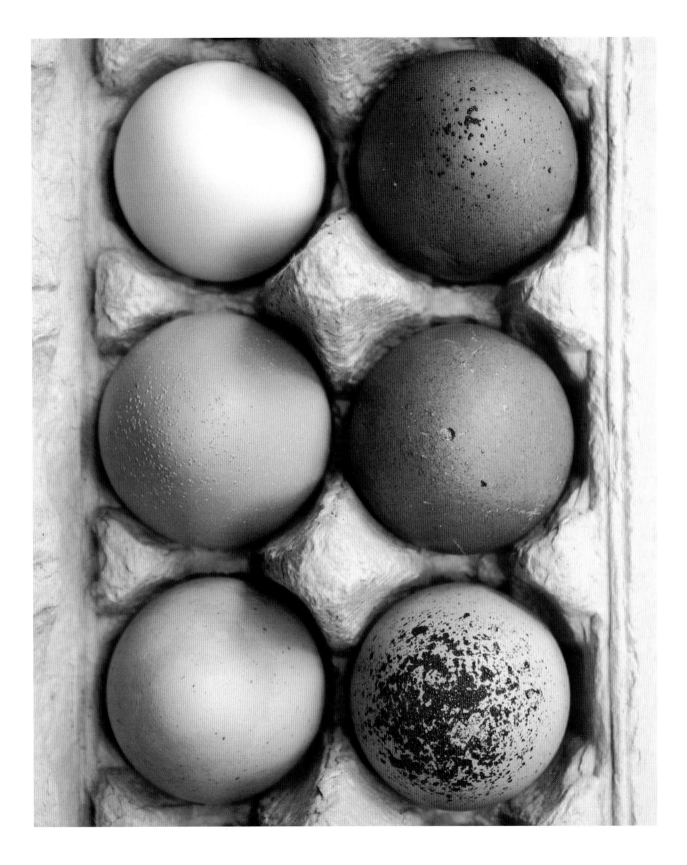

Breakfast

Blueberry and Bran Granola

vegan · vegetarian · dairy-free

Makes 4 cups

1 tablespoon canola oil

½ cup dried blueberries

½ cup finely chopped dried apples

½ cup chopped walnuts

1 tablespoon agave nectar

½ teaspoon ground cinnamon

½ teaspoon vanilla

2½ cups bran flakes

1. Preheat oven to 300°F. Brush 13×9-inch baking pan with oil.

2. Stir together blueberries, apples, walnuts, agave, cinnamon and vanilla in large bowl. Fold in bran flakes. Spread mixture in prepared pan.

3. Bake about 10 minutes or until mixture is browned and aromatic, stirring halfway through baking time. Cool completely before serving. Store in tightly covered container.

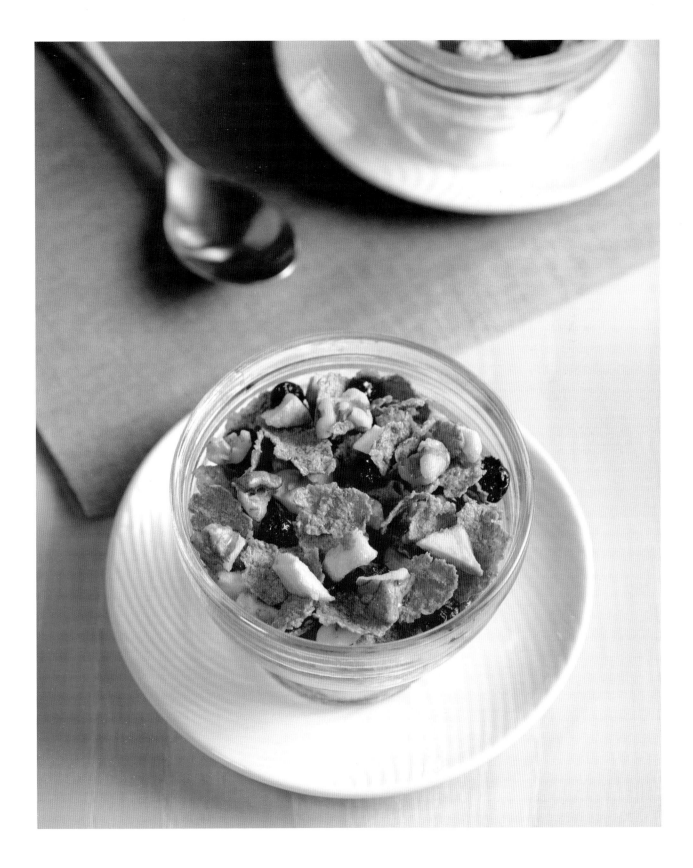

Pea and Spinach Frittata

vegetarian · **nut-free** · **gluten-free**

Makes 4 servings

6 **egg whites**

2 **eggs**

½ **cup cooked brown rice**

¼ **cup Greek yogurt**

2 **tablespoons grated Romano or Parmesan cheese, plus additional for garnish**

1 **tablespoon chopped fresh mint** *or* **1 teaspoon dried mint**

½ **teaspoon salt**

¼ **teaspoon black pepper**

1 **cup chopped onion**

¼ **cup water**

1 **cup peas**

1 **cup packed fresh spinach**

1. Combine egg whites, eggs, rice, yogurt, 2 tablespoons cheese, mint, salt and pepper in medium bowl.

2. Combine onion and water in large skillet. Bring to a boil over high heat. Reduce heat to medium; cover and cook 2 to 3 minutes or until onion is tender. Stir in peas; cook until heated through. Drain. Add spinach; cook and stir 1 minute or until spinach just begins to wilt.

3. Add egg mixture. Cook 2 minutes without stirring until eggs begin to set. Lift edge of eggs with spatula to allow uncooked portion to flow underneath. Remove skillet from heat when eggs are almost set but surface is still moist.

4. Cover and let stand 3 to 4 minutes or until surface is set. Sprinkle with additional cheese, if desired. Cut into four wedges to serve.

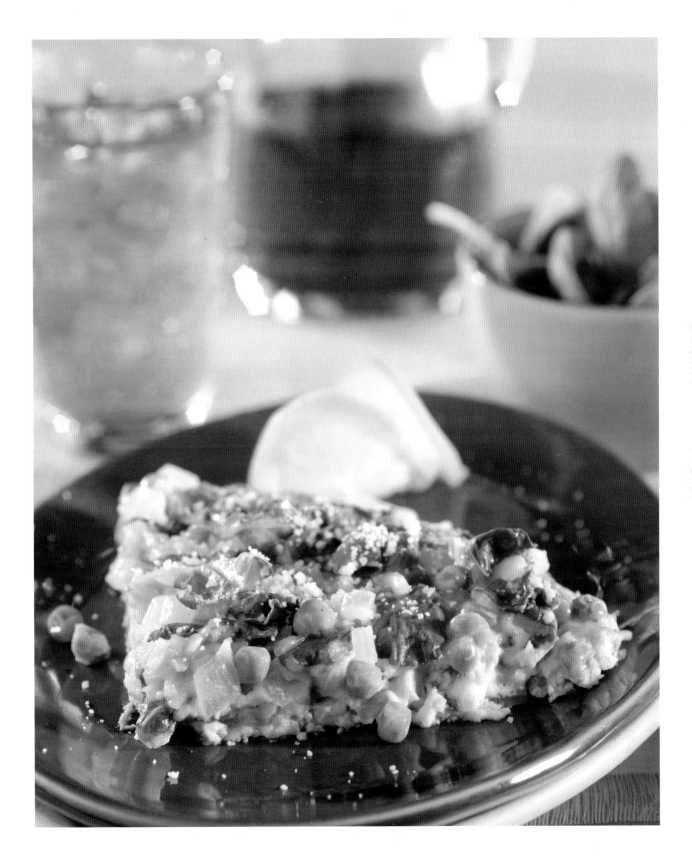

Overnight Oatmeal

vegan · vegetarian · dairy-free · gluten-free

Makes 6 servings

3 cups water

2 cups chopped peeled apples

1½ cups steel-cut or old-fashioned oats

¼ cup sliced almonds

½ teaspoon ground cinnamon

1. Combine water, apples, oats, almonds and cinnamon in slow cooker.

2. Cover; cook on LOW 8 hours.

Serving Suggestions: Top with sliced apples, maple syrup, agave nectar or turbinado sugar and/or dairy-free milk.

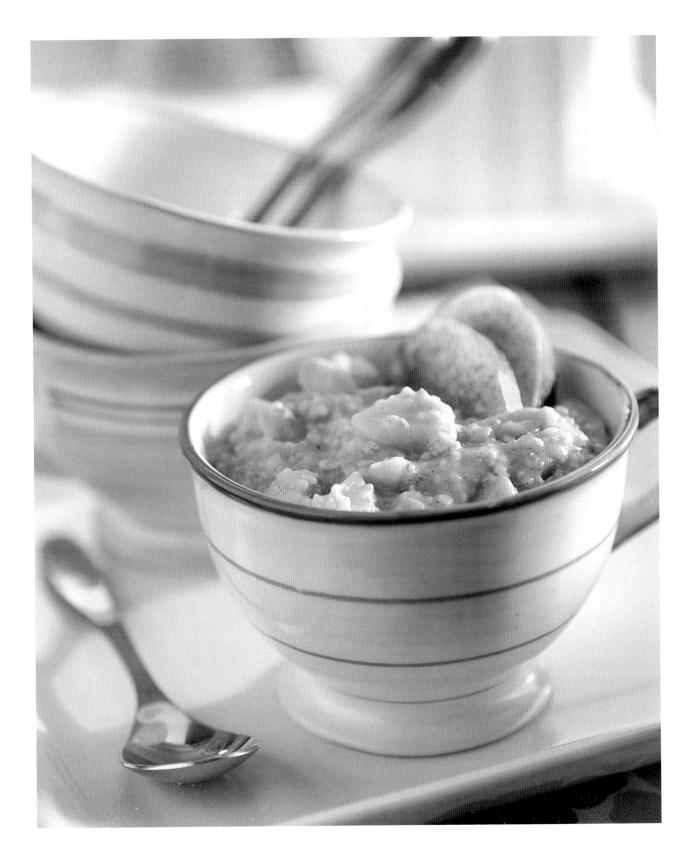

Vegan Pancakes

vegan · vegetarian · dairy-free · nut-free

Makes about 14 pancakes

- 2 **cups soymilk or other dairy-free milk**
- 2 **tablespoons fresh lemon juice**
- 2 **tablespoons canola oil**
- 1 **tablespoon agave nectar**
- 1 **cup all-purpose flour**
- 1 **cup spelt flour**
- 1 **teaspoon baking soda**
- 1 **teaspoon baking powder**
- ½ **teaspoon salt**
- 1 **to 2 tablespoons coconut oil, melted**
  Fresh fruit and/or maple syrup

1. Combine soymilk and lemon juice in large measuring cup or medium bowl; let stand 5 minutes. Stir in oil and agave.

2. Whisk all-purpose flour, spelt flour, baking soda, baking powder and salt in large bowl. Whisk in soymilk mixture until blended but still lumpy.

3. Heat large nonstick skillet or griddle over medium-high heat. Brush lightly with coconut oil. Pour batter into skillet in 4-inch circles. Cook 3 to 5 minutes or until edges are dull and bubbles appear on tops. Turn and cook 1 to 2 minutes or until browned. Keep warm.

4. Serve with fresh fruit or maple syrup.

Tip: To keep pancakes warm, place in a single layer on a wire rack in a 200°F oven.

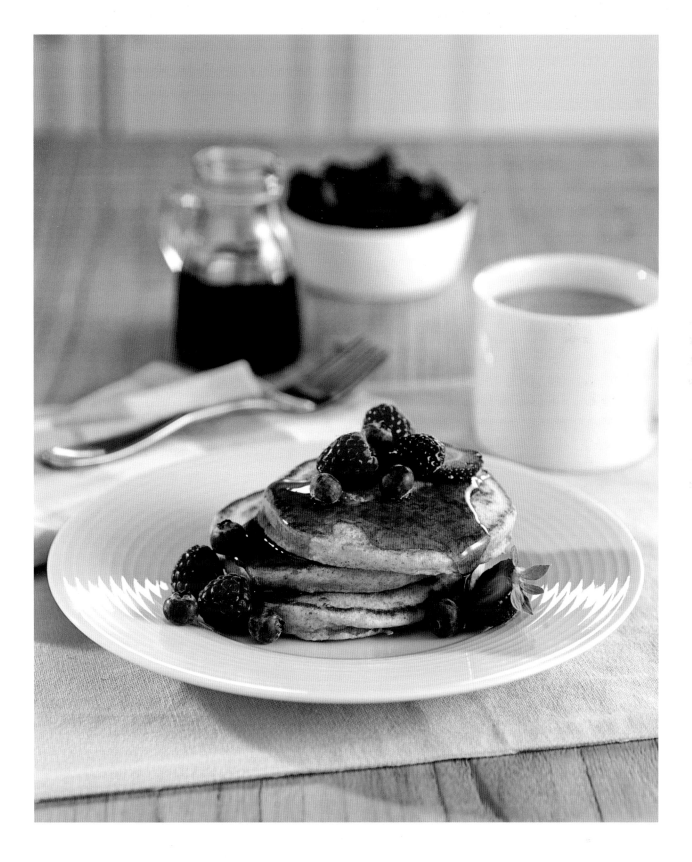

Oatmeal with Maple-Glazed Apples

vegan · vegetarian · dairy-free · nut-free · gluten-free

Makes 4 servings

3 cups water

¼ teaspoon salt

2 cups old-fashioned oats

1 teaspoon coconut oil

¼ teaspoon ground cinnamon

2 medium unpeeled apples,
    cut into ½-inch chunks

2 tablespoons maple syrup

¼ cup dried cranberries

1. Bring water and salt to a boil in large saucepan. Stir in oats. Reduce heat; simmer 5 to 6 minutes, stirring occasionally.

2. Meanwhile, melt coconut oil in large nonstick skillet over medium heat; stir in cinnamon. Add apples; cook and stir 4 to 5 minutes or until tender. Stir in maple syrup.

3. Spoon oatmeal into four bowls; top with apple mixture and cranberries

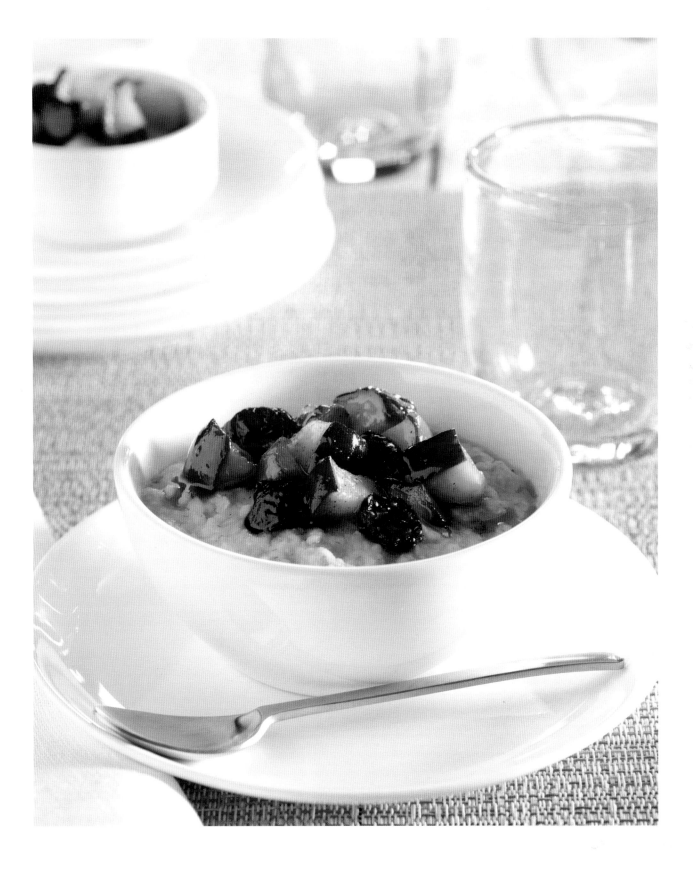

Scrambled Tofu and Potatoes

vegan • vegetarian • dairy-free • nut-free • gluten-free

Makes 4 servings

Potatoes

- ¼ **cup extra virgin olive oil**
- 4 **red potatoes, cubed**
- ½ **white onion, sliced**
- 1 **tablespoon chopped fresh rosemary**
- 1 **teaspoon coarse salt**

Scrambled Tofu

- ¼ **cup nutritional yeast**
- ½ **teaspoon ground turmeric**
- 2 **tablespoons water**
- 2 **tablespoons tamari**
- 1 **package (14 ounces) firm tofu**
- 2 **teaspoons extra virgin olive oil**
- ½ **cup chopped green bell pepper**
- ½ **cup chopped red onion**

1. For potatoes, preheat oven to 450°F. Add ¼ cup olive oil to 12-inch cast iron skillet; place skillet in oven 10 minutes to heat.

2. Bring large saucepan of water to a boil. Add potatoes; cook 5 to 7 minutes or until tender. Drain potatoes and return to saucepan; stir in white onion, rosemary and salt. Spread mixture in preheated skillet. Bake 25 to 30 minutes or until potatoes are browned, stirring every 10 minutes.

3. For tofu, combine nutritional yeast and turmeric in small bowl. Stir in water and tamari until smooth.

4. Cut tofu into large cubes. Gently squeeze out water; loosely crumble tofu into medium bowl. Heat 2 teaspoons olive oil in large skillet over medium-high heat. Add bell pepper and red onion; cook and stir 2 minutes or until soft but not browned. Add tofu; drizzle with 3 tablespoons nutritional yeast sauce. Cook and stir about 5 minutes or until liquid is evaporated and tofu is heated through. Stir in additional sauce for stronger flavor, if desired.

5. Divide potatoes among four serving plates; top with tofu.

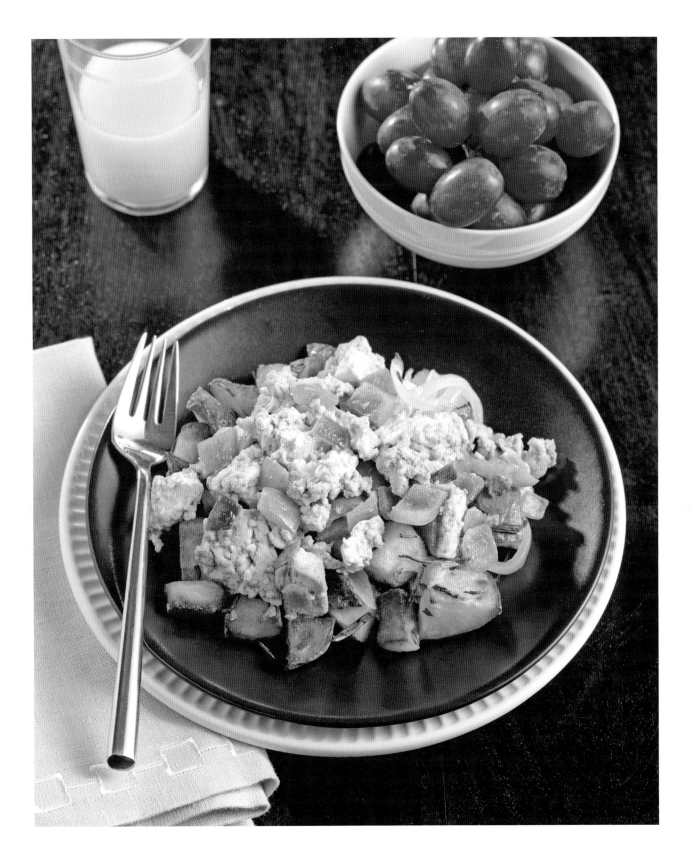

Banana Split Breakfast Bowl

vegetarian · gluten-free

Makes 4 servings

- 3 **tablespoons sliced almonds**
- 3 **tablespoons chopped walnuts**
- 3 **cups plain yogurt**
- 1 **cup sliced fresh strawberries**
- 2 **bananas, cut into quarters**
- ½ **cup fresh pineapple chunks or drained canned pineapple tidbits**

1. Spread almonds and walnuts in single layer in small heavy skillet. Cook and stir over medium heat 2 minutes or until lightly browned. Immediately remove from skillet; cool completely.

2. Spoon yogurt into four serving bowls. Top with strawberries, bananas and pineapple. Sprinkle with toasted nuts.

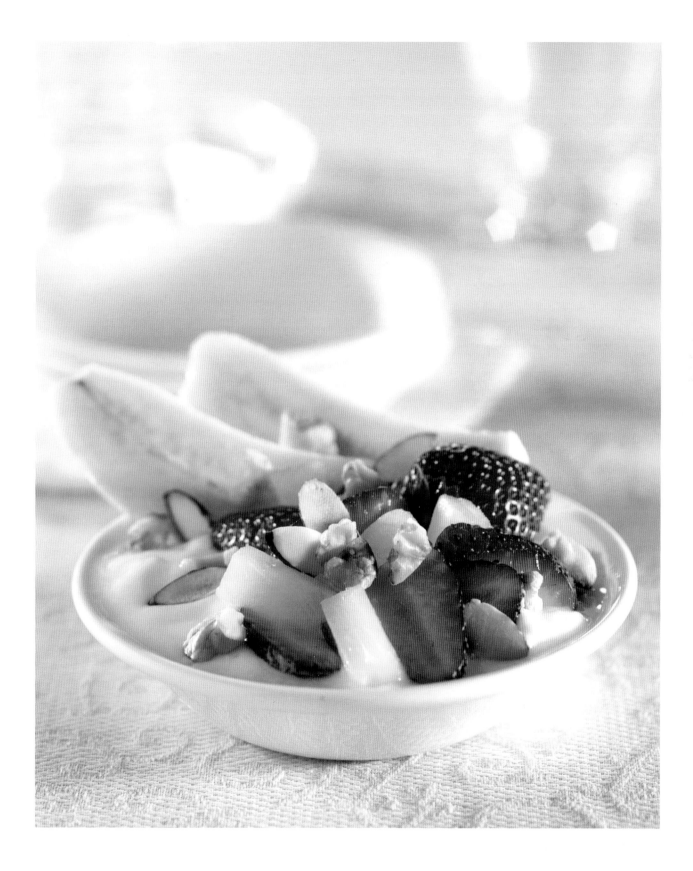

Date-Nut Granola

vegetarian · dairy-free

Makes 6 cups

⅓ cup plus 1 tablespoon
   canola oil, divided
2 cups old-fashioned oats
2 cups barley flakes
1 cup sliced almonds
⅓ cup honey
1 teaspoon vanilla
1 cup chopped dates

1. Preheat oven to 350°F. Brush 13×9-inch baking pan with 1 tablespoon oil.

2. Combine oats, barley flakes and almonds in large bowl. Combine remaining ⅓ cup oil, honey and vanilla in small bowl; mix well. Pour over oat mixture; stir until well blended. Spread in prepared pan.

3. Bake about 25 minutes or until toasted, stirring frequently after 10 minutes. Stir in dates while granola is still hot. Cool. Store in airtight container.

Variation: To make this recipe vegan, replace honey with agave nectar or maple syrup.

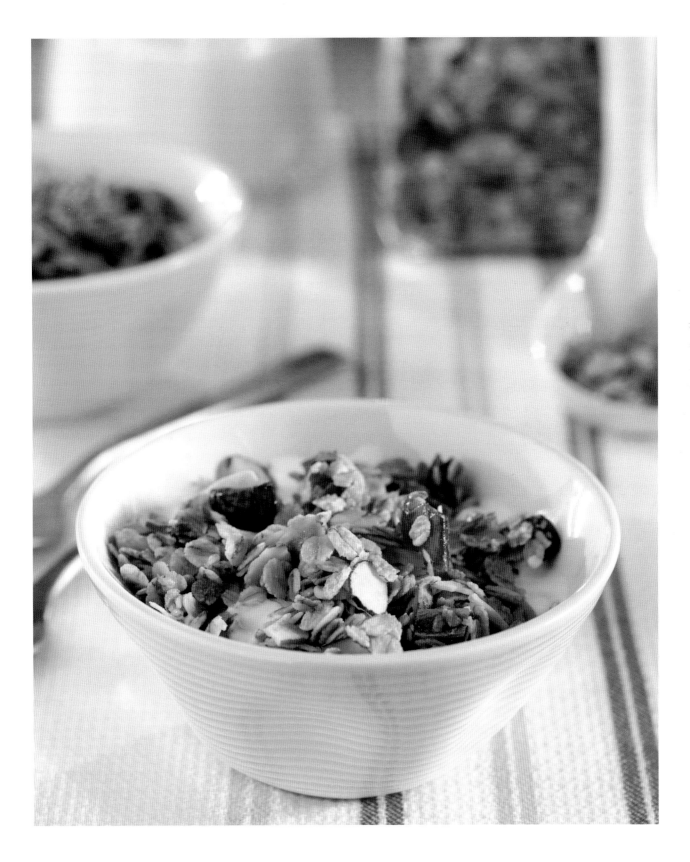

Zucchini Omelet with Dill

vegetarian · nut-free · gluten-free

Makes 2 servings

4 **egg whites**

1 **whole egg**

2 **tablespoons milk**

½ **teaspoon dried dill weed**

⅛ **teaspoon coarse salt**

⅛ **teaspoon black pepper**

1 **teaspoon butter**

1 **cup finely diced zucchini**

1. Whisk egg white, whole egg, milk, dill, salt and pepper in medium bowl until blended.

2. Melt butter in medium skillet over medium-high heat. Add zucchini; cook 4 minutes or until lightly browned, stirring occasionally.

3. Add egg mixture and cook until edges are set. Lift edge of egg mixture with spatula to allow uncooked portion to flow underneath. When eggs are set, fold omelet over. Cut in half; serve immediately.

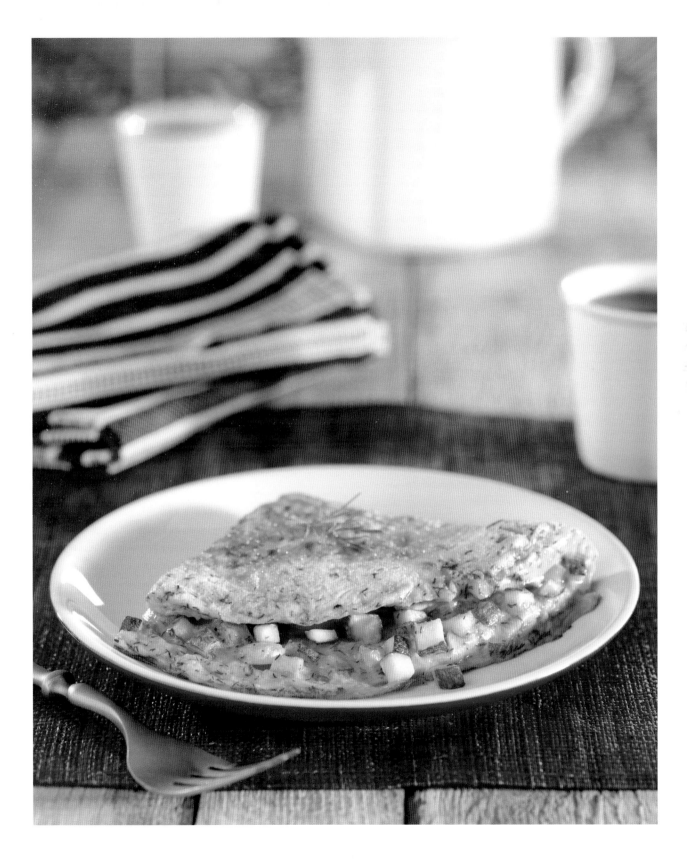

Apple-Raspberry Granola Skillet

vegetarian · dairy-free

Makes 8 servings

---

1 cup granola without raisins

2 tablespoons water

1 tablespoon fresh lemon juice

2 teaspoons cornstarch

1 pound apples, cored and sliced

½ teaspoon ground cinnamon

4 ounces frozen raspberries

1 tablespoon honey

½ teaspoon vanilla

¼ teaspoon almond extract

1. Place granola in small resealable food storage bag; seal bag. Crush with rolling pin or meat mallet until coarse crumbs form; set aside.

2. Combine water, lemon juice and cornstarch in small bowl; stir until cornstarch is dissolved.

3. Combine apples, cornstarch mixture and cinnamon in medium skillet; stir until blended. Bring to a boil over medium-high heat. Boil 1 minute or until thickened, stirring constantly.

4. Remove skillet from heat. Gently fold in raspberries, honey, vanilla and almond extract. Sprinkle granola crumbs evenly over top. Let stand, uncovered, 30 minutes.

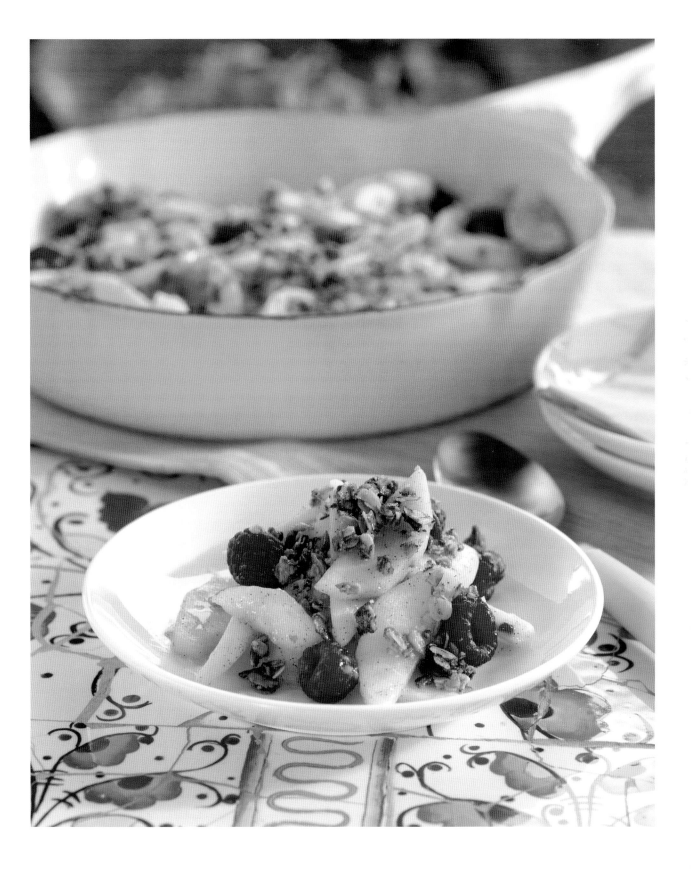

Edamame Frittata

vegetarian · nut-free · gluten-free

Makes 4 servings

2 **tablespoons olive oil**

½ **cup shelled edamame**

⅓ **cup corn**

¼ **cup chopped shallot**

5 **eggs**

¾ **teaspoon dried Italian seasoning**

½ **teaspoon salt**

½ **teaspoon black pepper**

¼ **cup chopped green onions**

½ **cup crumbled goat cheese**

1. Preheat broiler. Heat oil in large ovenproof skillet over medium-high heat. Add edamame, corn and shallot; cook and stir 6 to 8 minutes or until shallot is browned and edamame are hot.

2. Meanwhile, beat eggs, seasoning, salt and pepper in medium bowl. Stir in green onions. Pour egg mixture over vegetables in skillet. Sprinkle with cheese. Cook over medium heat 5 to 7 minutes or until eggs are set on bottom, lifting edge of eggs to allow uncooked portion to flow underneath.

3. Broil 6 inches from heat 1 minute or until top is puffed and golden. Loosen frittata from skillet with spatula; slide onto cutting board. Cut into wedges.

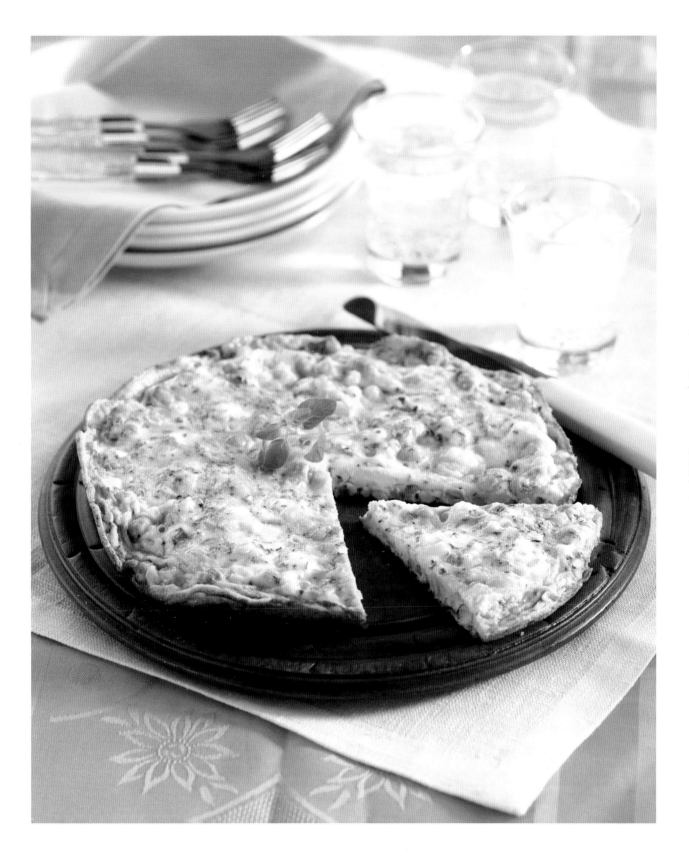

Melon Cup

Makes 4 servings

2 **cups cubed watermelon or any melon**

2 **cups plain yogurt**

½ **cup natural granola**

Divide melon among four serving dishes. Top with yogurt and granola.

Variation: To make this recipe vegan, substitute soy yogurt or coconut yogurt for the plain yogurt.

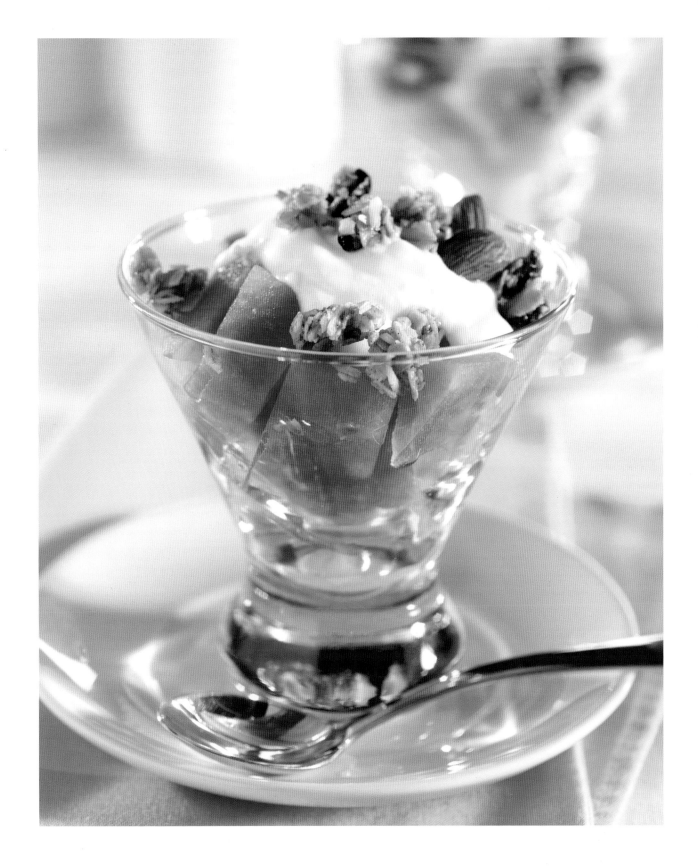

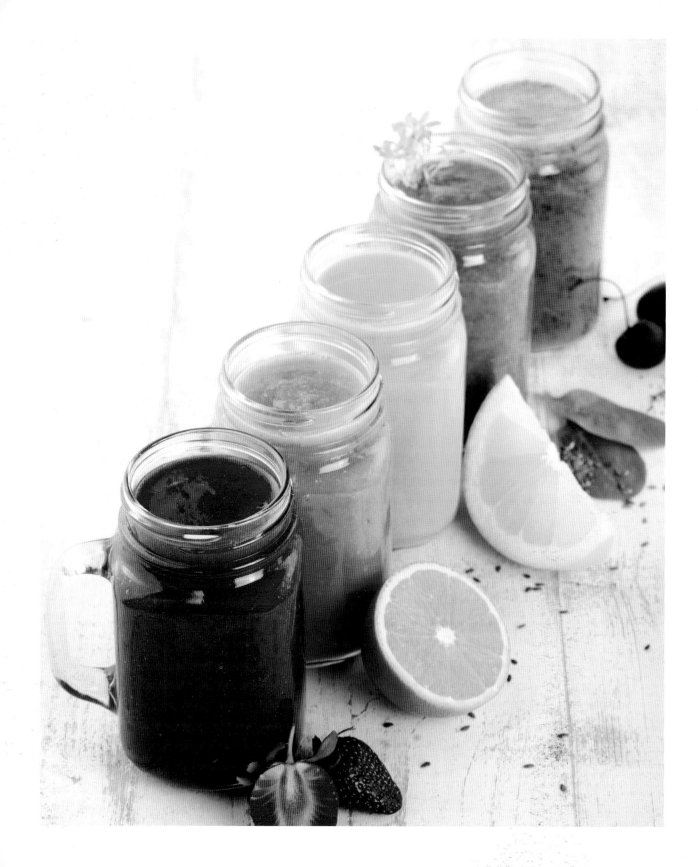

Juices & Smoothies

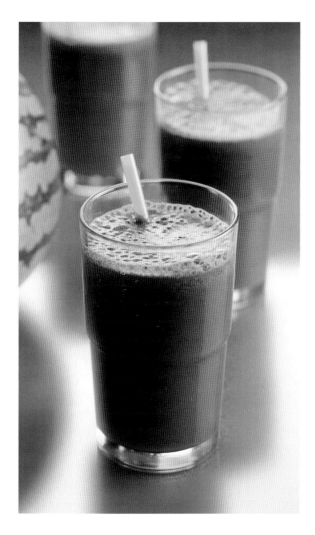

Super C Juice

Makes 3 servings

- **2 oranges, peeled**
- **1 grapefruit, peeled**
- **1 lemon, peeled**
- **½ cup fresh or frozen cranberries**
- **2 teaspoons honey**

Juice oranges, grapefruit, lemon and cranberries. Stir in honey until blended.

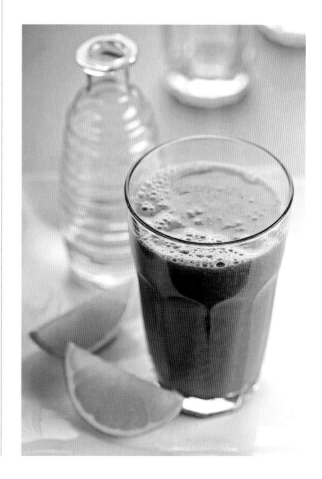

Melonade

Makes 4 servings

- **¼ seedless watermelon, rind removed**
- **1 apple**
- **1 lemon, peeled**

Juice watermelon, apple and lemon. Stir.

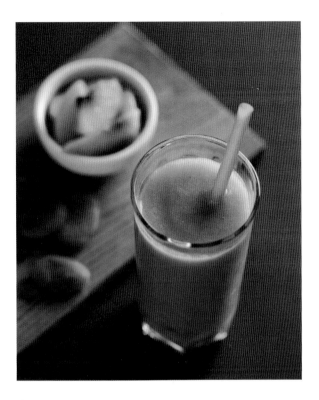

Peach Apricot Smoothie

vegan · vegetarian · dairy-free · **nut-free** · **gluten-free**

Makes 2 servings

- ½ **cup dried apricots**
- ¼ **cup water**
- ¼ **cup fresh orange juice**
- 1 **cup frozen sliced peaches**
- ¼ **teaspoon ground ginger**

1. Place apricots in small bowl; cover with hot water. Let stand 20 minutes or until soft; drain.

2. Combine ¼ cup water, orange juice, peaches, apricots and ginger in blender; blend until smooth. Serve immediately.

Morning Juice Blend

vegan · vegetarian · dairy-free · **nut-free** · **gluten-free**

Makes 2 servings

- ¼ **pineapple, peeled**
- 1 **orange, peeled**
- 1 **inch fresh ginger, peeled**

Juice pineapple, orange and ginger. Stir.

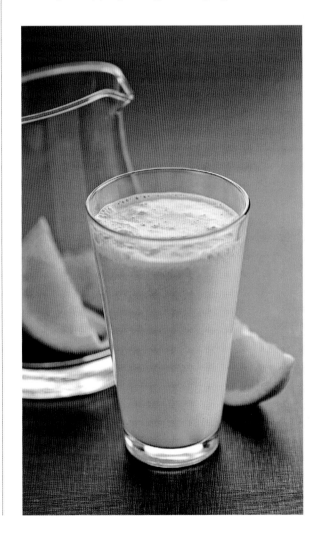

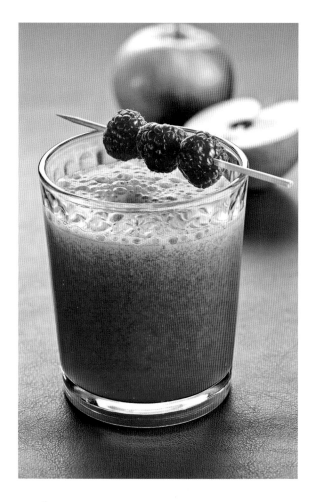

Orange Apricot Sunshine Smoothie

vegan · vegetarian · dairy-free · nut-free · gluten-free

Makes 2 servings

- ½ **cup dried apricots**
- ¾ **cup water**
- 1 **orange, peeled and seeded**
- ½ **cup frozen mango chunks**
- ½ **teaspoon grated fresh ginger**

Place apricots in small bowl; cover with hot water. Let stand 20 minutes; drain. Combine ¾ cup water, orange, mango, apricots and ginger in blender; blend until smooth. Serve immediately.

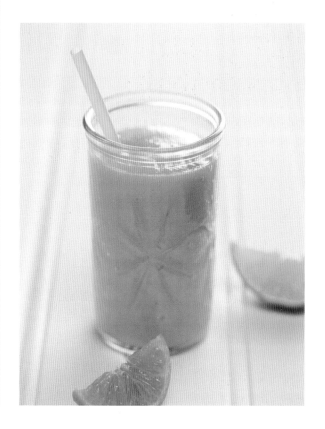

Red Orange Juice

vegan · vegetarian · dairy-free · nut-free · gluten-free

Makes 2 servings

- 1 **orange, peeled**
- 1 **apple**
- ½ **cup fresh raspberries**
- ½ **cup stemmed strawberries**

Juice orange, apple, raspberries and strawberries. Stir.

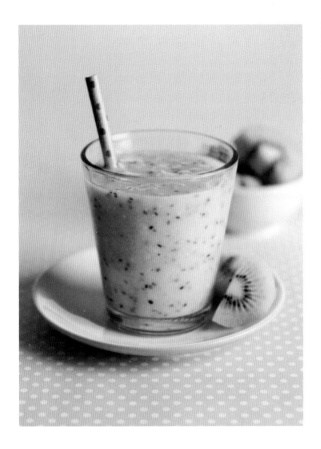

Kiwi Green Dream

vegan · vegetarian · dairy-free · nut-free · gluten-free

Makes 2 servings

- ¾ **cup water**
- 2 **kiwis, peeled and quartered**
- ½ **cup frozen pineapple chunks**
- ½ **avocado**
- 1 **tablespoon chia seeds**

Combine water, kiwis, pineapple and avocado in blender; blend until smooth. Add chia seeds; blend until smooth. Serve immediately.

Red Cabbage and Pineapple Juice

vegan · vegetarian · dairy-free · nut-free · **gluten-free**

Makes 2 servings

- ¼ **red cabbage**
- ¼ **pineapple, peeled**

Juice cabbage and pineapple. Stir.

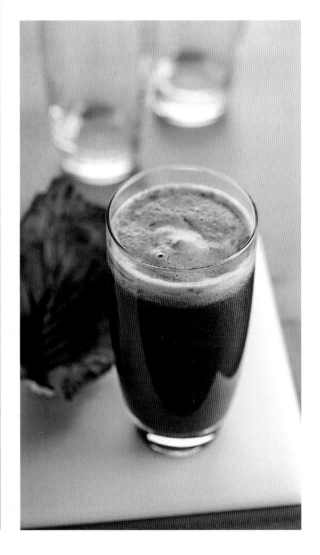

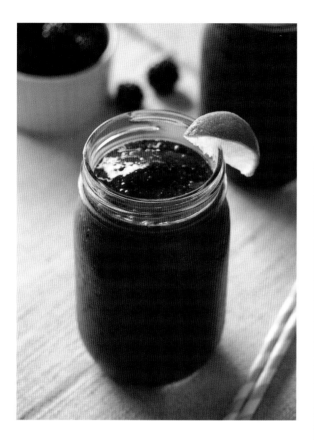

Blackberry Lime Smoothie

vegetarian · dairy-free · nut-free · gluten-free

Makes 1 serving

- ½ **cup unsweetened coconut milk**
- 1 **cup fresh blackberries**
- 2 **ice cubes**
- 1 **tablespoon fresh lime juice**
- 2 **teaspoons honey**
- ½ **teaspoon grated lime peel**

Combine coconut milk, blackberries, ice, lime juice, honey and lime peel in blender; blend until smooth. Serve immediately.

Sweet Green Supreme

vegan · vegetarian · dairy-free · nut-free · gluten-free

Makes 2 servings

- 2 **cups seedless green grapes**
- ½ **frozen banana**
- ½ **cup baby kale**
- ½ **cup ice cubes**

Combine grapes, banana, kale and ice in blender; blend until smooth. Serve immediately.

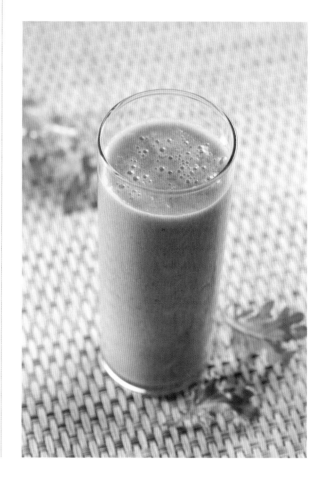

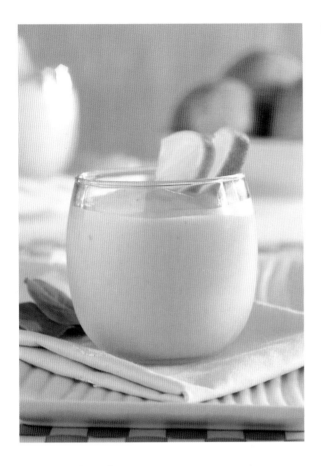

Mango Madness

vegan · vegetarian · dairy-free · **gluten-free**

Makes 2 servings

- ½ **cup water**
- ½ **cup unsweetened almond milk**
- 1 **cup frozen mango chunks**
- ½ **cup frozen sliced peaches**
- ½ **banana**

Combine water, almond milk, mango, peaches and banana in blender; blend until smooth. Serve immediately.

Sweet Beet Treat

vegan · **vegetarian** · dairy-free · **nut-free** · **gluten-free**

Makes 2 servings

- ¼ **cup water**
- 2 **medium carrots, cut into chunks (about 4 ounces)**
- 1 **medium beet, peeled and cut into chunks**
- 1 **large sweet red apple, seeded and cut into chunks**
- ¼ **cup ice cubes**
- 1 **tablespoon fresh lemon juice**

Combine water, carrots, beet, apple, ice and lemon juice in blender; blend until smooth. Serve immediately.

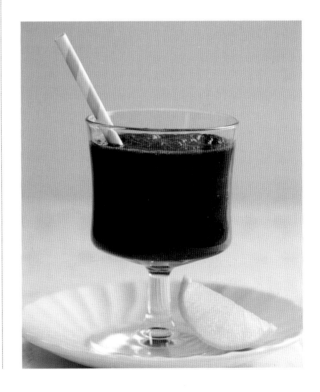

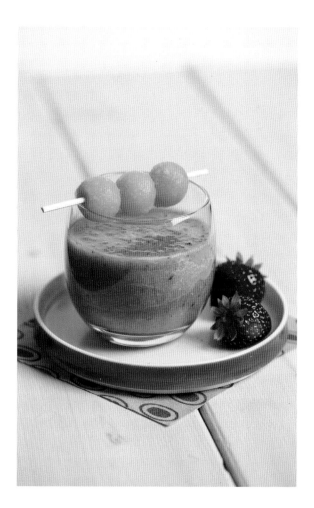

Raspberry Cherry Smoothie

vegan · vegetarian · dairy-free · nut-free · gluten-free

Makes 2 servings

- ⅔ **cup apple juice**
- 1 **cup frozen raspberries**
- 1 **cup frozen dark sweet cherries, slightly thawed**
- ½ **avocado**

Combine apple juice, raspberries, cherries and avocado in blender; blend until smooth. Serve immediately.

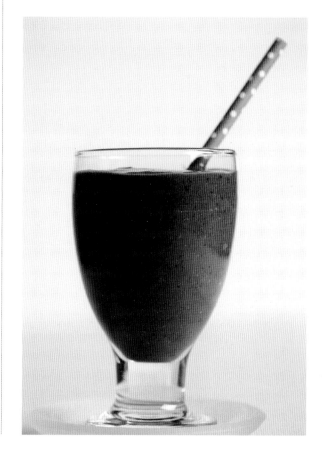

Cantaloupe Strawberry Sunrise

vegan · vegetarian · dairy-free · nut-free · gluten-free

Makes 2 servings

- 1 **cup cantaloupe chunks**
- 2 **clementines, peeled**
- 1 **cup frozen strawberries**

Combine cantaloupe, clementines and strawberries in blender; blend until smooth. Serve immediately.

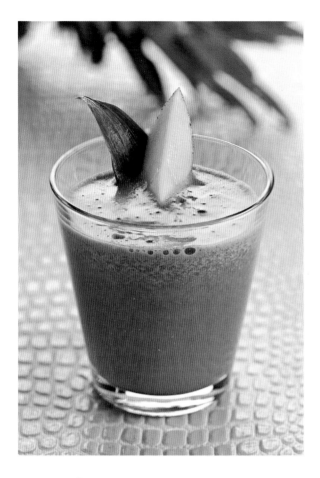

Tropical Twist Juice

vegan · vegetarian · dairy-free · nut-free · gluten-free

Makes 2 servings

⅛ **pineapple, peeled**
⅛ **seedless watermelon, rind removed**
1 **orange, peeled**
½ **mango, peeled**
⅓ **cup stemmed strawberries**

Juice pineapple, watermelon, orange, mango and strawberries. Stir.

Energizing Juice

vegan · vegetarian · dairy-free · nut-free · gluten-free

Makes 2 servings

2 **tomatoes**
½ **cucumber**
8 **green beans**
½ **lemon, peeled**
Dash hot pepper sauce

Juice tomatoes, cucumber, green beans and lemon. Stir in hot pepper sauce until well blended.

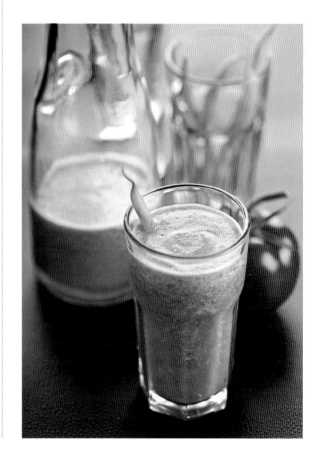

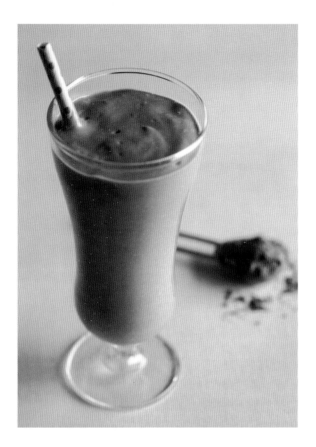

Blueberry Apple Juice

vegan · vegetarian · dairy-free · nut-free · gluten-free

Makes 2 servings

- 2 **apples**
- 1½ **cups fresh blueberries**
- ½ **grapefruit, peeled**
- 1 **inch fresh ginger, peeled**

Juice apples, blueberries, grapefruit and ginger. Stir.

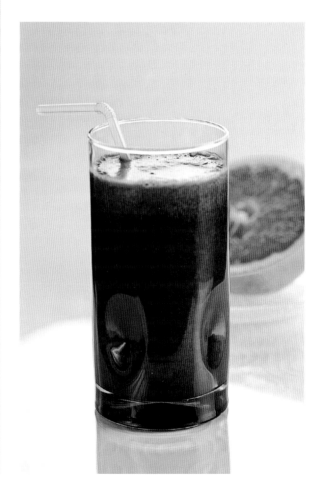

Creamy Chocolate Smoothie

vegetarian · dairy-free · gluten-free

Makes 1 serving

- 1 **cup unsweetened almond milk**
- 1 **frozen banana**
- ½ **avocado**
- 1 **tablespoon unsweetened cocoa powder**
- 1 **tablespoon honey**

Combine almond milk, banana, avocado, cocoa and honey in blender; blend until smooth. Serve immediately.

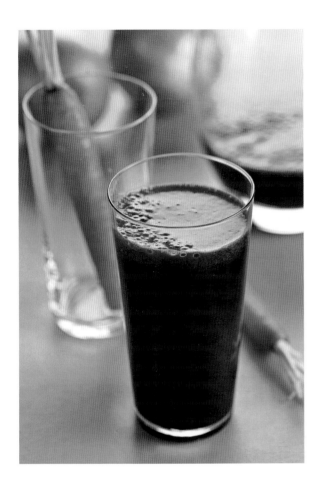

Cleansing Green Juice

vegan · vegetarian · dairy-free · nut-free · gluten-free

Makes 2 servings

- 4 **leaves bok choy**
- 1 **stalk celery**
- ½ **cucumber**
- ¼ **bulb fennel**
- ½ **lemon, peeled**

Juice bok choy, celery, cucumber, fennel and lemon. Stir.

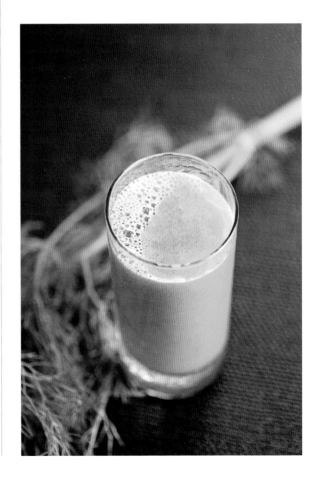

Veggie Delight Juice

vegan · vegetarian · dairy-free · nut-free · gluten-free

Makes 2 servings

- 1 **carrot**
- 1 **stalk celery**
- 1 **beet**
- 1 **apple**
- ½ **small sweet onion**

Juice carrot, celery, beet, apple and onion. Stir.

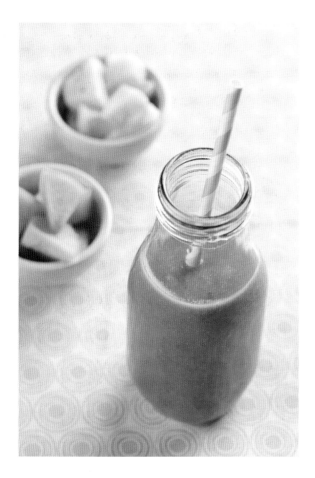

Triple Pepper Juice

vegan · vegetarian · dairy-free · nut-free · gluten-free

Makes 2 servings

> 2 **apples**
> 1 **red bell pepper**
> 1 **yellow bell pepper**
> ½ **jalapeño pepper**

Juice apples, bell peppers and jalapeño pepper. Stir.

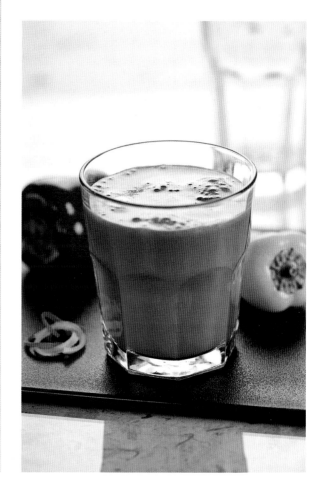

Green Cantaloupe Quencher

vegan · vegetarian · dairy-free · nut-free · gluten-free

Makes 2 servings

> 2 **cups cantaloupe chunks**
> 1 **cup frozen pineapple chunks**
> 1 **cup baby spinach**
> 1 **tablespoon ground flaxseed**

Combine cantaloupe, pineapple, spinach and flaxseed in blender; blend until smooth. Serve immediately.

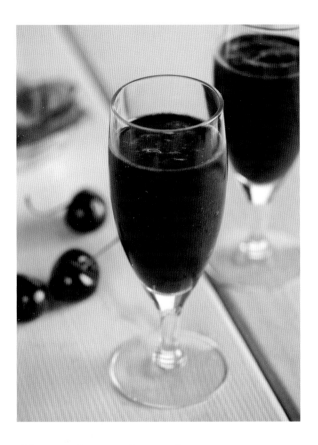

Strawberry Clementine Smoothie

vegan · vegetarian · dairy-free · nut-free · gluten-free

Makes 2 servings

- ⅓ **cup water**
- 2 **cups frozen strawberries, slightly thawed**
- 1 **frozen banana**
- 2 **clementines, peeled**

Combine water, strawberries, banana and clemetines in blender; blend until smooth. Serve immediately.

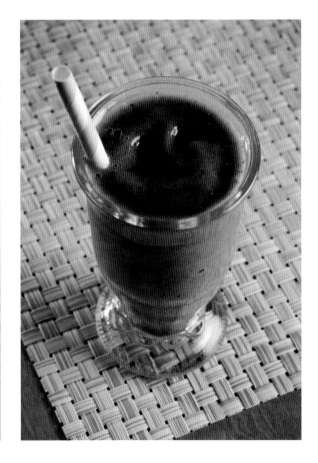

Cherry Green Smoothie

vegetarian · dairy-free · **gluten-free**

Makes 2 servings

- ¾ **cup almond milk**
- 1½ **cups frozen dark sweet cherries**
- ¾ **cup baby spinach**
- ½ **frozen banana**
- 1 **tablespoon ground flaxseed**
- 2 **teaspoons honey**

Combine almond milk, cherries, spinach, banana, flaxseed and honey in blender; blend until smooth. Serve immediately.

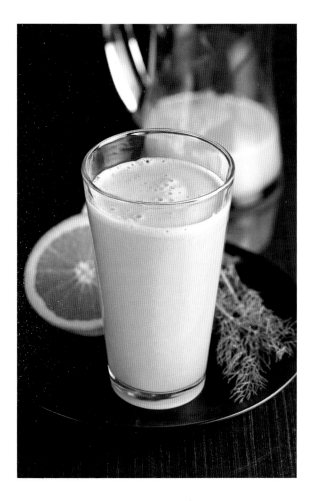

Super Citrus Smoothie

vegetarian · dairy-free · nut-free · gluten-free

Makes 3 servings

- ⅔ **cup water**
- 2 **oranges, peeled and seeded**
- 2 **cups frozen blackberries**
- 2 **cups baby kale**
- 1 **avocado**
- 2 **tablespoons honey**

Combine water, oranges, blackberries, kale, avocado and honey in blender; blend until smooth. Serve immediately.

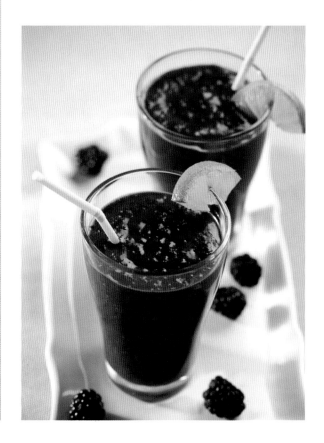

Orange Fennel Sprout Juice

vegan · vegetarian · dairy-free · nut-free · gluten-free

Makes 2 servings

- 2 **oranges, peeled**
- 2 **stalks celery**
- 1 **bulb fennel**
- 1 **cup alfalfa sprouts**

Juice oranges, celery, fennel and alfalfa sprouts. Stir.

Apple, Sweet Potato and Carrot Juice

vegan · vegetarian · dairy-free · nut-free · gluten-free

Makes 4 servings

4 apples
1 sweet potato
1 carrot

Juice apples, sweet potato and carrot. Stir.

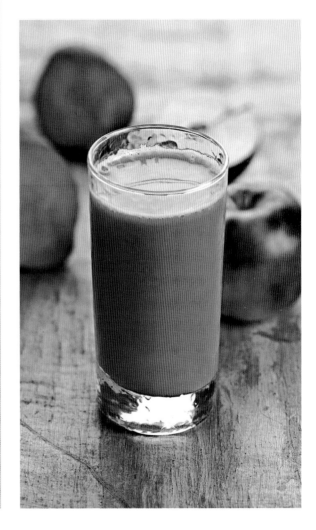

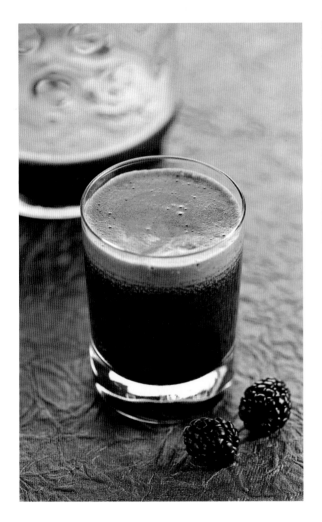

Immunity Booster

vegan · vegetarian · dairy-free · nut-free · gluten-free

Makes 3 servings

1 grapefruit, peeled
2 oranges, peeled
½ cup fresh blackberries

Juice grapefruit, oranges and blackberries. Stir.

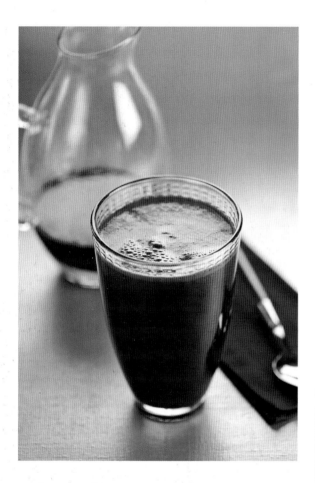

Super Blue Smoothie
vegetarian · dairy-free · nut-free · gluten-free

Makes 2 servings

- ½ **cup pomegranate juice**
- ¼ **cup water**
- ¾ **cup frozen blueberries**
- ¾ **cup frozen blackberries**
- ½ **avocado**
- 2 **teaspoons honey**

Combine pomegranate juice, water, blueberries, blackberries, avocado and honey in blender; blend until smooth.

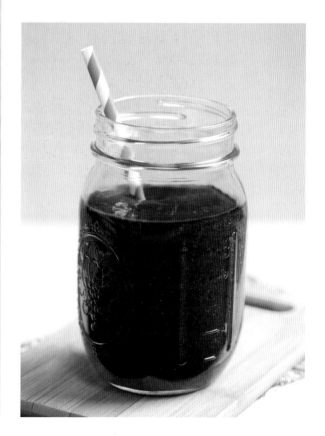

Ruby Apple Stinger
vegan · vegetarian · dairy-free · nut-free · gluten-free

Makes 2 servings

- 2 **beets**
- 2 **carrots**
- ½ **apple**
- 1 **inch fresh ginger, peeled**
- ¼ **lemon, peeled**

Juice beets, carrots, apple, ginger and lemon. Stir.

Triple Green Smoothie

vegan · vegetarian · dairy-free · **nut-free** · **gluten-free**

Makes 2 servings

   2 cups seedless green grapes
   1 kiwi, peeled and quartered
   ½ avocado

Combine grapes, kiwi and avocado in blender; blend until smooth. Serve immediately.

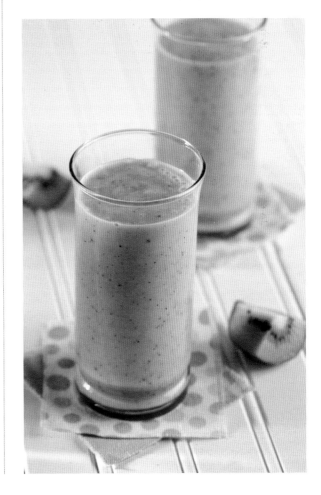

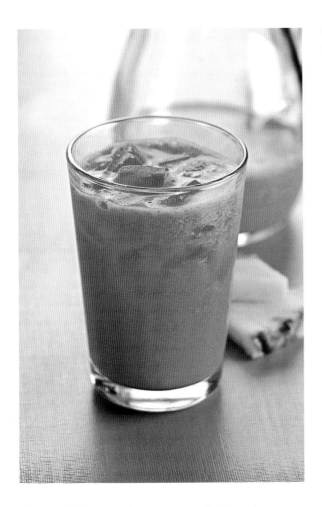

Spicy Pineapple Carrot Juice

vegan · vegetarian · dairy-free · **nut-free** · **gluten-free**

Makes 2 servings

   ½ pineapple, peeled
   2 carrots
   1 inch fresh ginger, peeled
   Ice cubes

Juice pineapple, carrots and ginger. Stir. Serve over ice.

Tangy Apple Kale Smoothie

vegan · vegetarian · dairy-free · nut-free · gluten-free

Makes 3 servings

- 1 **cup water**
- 2 **Granny Smith apples, seeded and cut into chunks**
- 2 **cups baby kale**
- 1 **frozen banana**

Combine water, apples, kale and banana in blender; blend until smooth. Serve immediately.

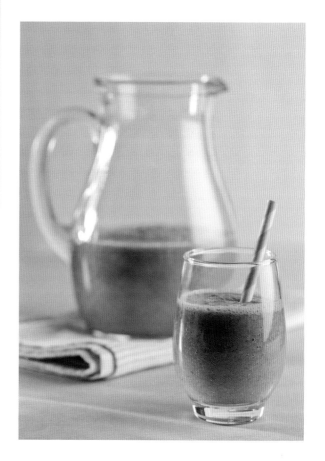

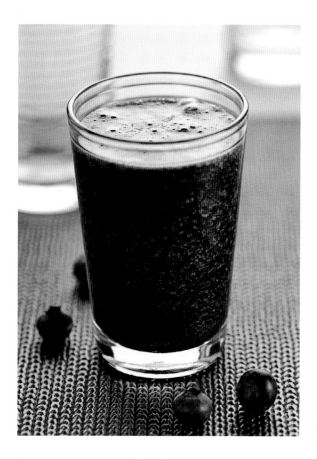

Super Berry Refresher

vegan · vegetarian · dairy-free · nut-free · glut n-free

Makes 2 servings

- 1 **cup stemmed fresh strawberries**
- 1 **cup fresh raspberries**
- 1 **cucumber**
- ½ **cup fresh blackberries**
- ½ **cup fresh blueberries**
- ¼ **lemon, peeled**

Juice strawberries, raspberries, cucumber, blackberries, blueberries and lemon. Stir.

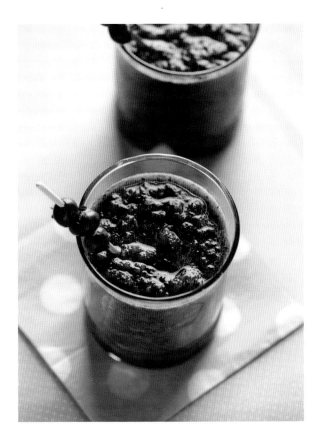

Cantaloupe Smoothie

vegan · vegetarian · dairy-free · **nut-free** · **gluten-free**

Makes 1 serving

- ½ **cup fresh orange juice**
- 2 **cups cantaloupe chunks**
- ½ **cup ice cubes**
- ½ **teaspoon vanilla**

Combine orange juice, cantaloupe, ice and vanilla in blender; blend until smooth. Serve immediately.

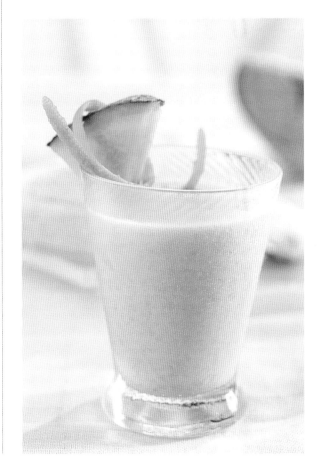

Blueberry Peach Bliss

vegan · vegetarian · dairy-free · **nut-free** · **gluten-free**

Makes 2 servings

- 1¼ **cups water**
- 1 **cup frozen blueberries**
- 1 **cup frozen sliced peaches**
- 1 **tablespoon fresh lemon juice**
- 2 **teaspoons agave nectar**
- ½ **teaspoon grated fresh ginger**

Combine water, blueberries, peaches, lemon juice, agave and ginger in blender; blend until smooth. Serve immediately.

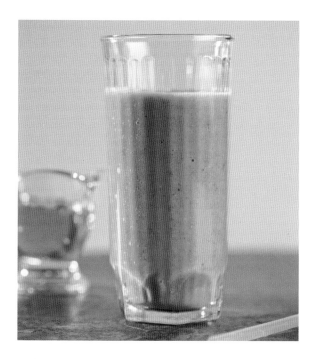

Spiced Pumpkin Banana Smoothie
vegetarian · dairy-free · **gluten-free**

Makes 1 serving

- ½ **cup almond milk**
- ½ **frozen banana**
- ½ **cup canned pumpkin**
- ½ **cup ice cubes**
- 1 **tablespoon honey**
- 1 **teaspoon ground flaxseed**
- ¼ **teaspoon ground cinnamon**
- ⅛ **teaspoon ground ginger**
- **Dash ground nutmeg**

Combine almond milk, banana, pumpkin, ice, honey, flaxseed, cinnamon, ginger and nutmeg in blender; blend until smooth. Serve immediately.

Cherry Berry Pomegranate Smoothie
vegan · **vegetarian** · dairy-free · **nut-free** · **gluten-free**

Makes 2 servings

- ¾ **cup water**
- 1 **cup frozen dark sweet cherries**
- ½ **cup frozen strawberries**
- ½ **cup pomegranate seeds**
- 1 **teaspoon fresh lemon juice**
- 1 **tablespoon chia seeds**

Combine water, cherries, strawberries, pomegranate seeds and lemon juice in blender; blend until smooth. Add chia seeds; blend until smooth. Serve immediately.

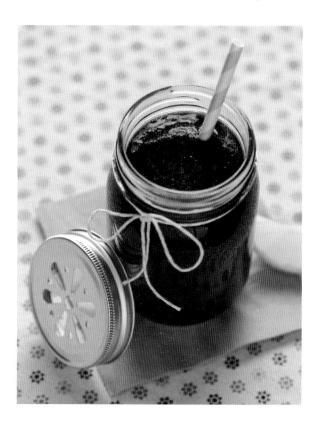

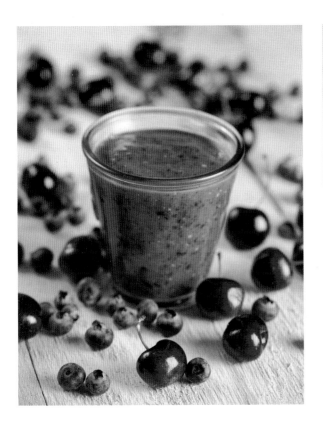

Tangerine Ginger Sipper
vegan · vegetarian · dairy-free · **nut-free** · **gluten-free**

Makes 2 servings

- 1 **tangerine, peeled**
- 1 **pear**
- ¼ **lemon, peeled**
- ½ **inch fresh ginger, peeled**

Juice tangerine, pear, lemon and ginger. Stir.

Blueberry Cherry Blend
vegan · vegetarian · dairy-free · **nut-free** · **gluten-free**

Makes 2 servings

- ¾ **cup water**
- ¾ **cup frozen blueberries**
- ¾ **cup frozen dark sweet cherries**
- ½ **avocado**
- 1 **tablespoon fresh lemon juice**
- 1 **teaspoon ground flaxseed**

Combine water, blueberries, cherries, avocado, lemon juice and flaxseed in blender; blend until smooth. Serve immediately.

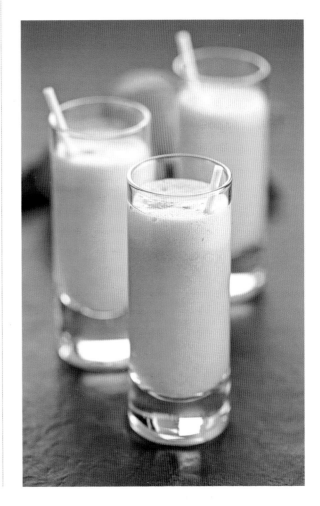

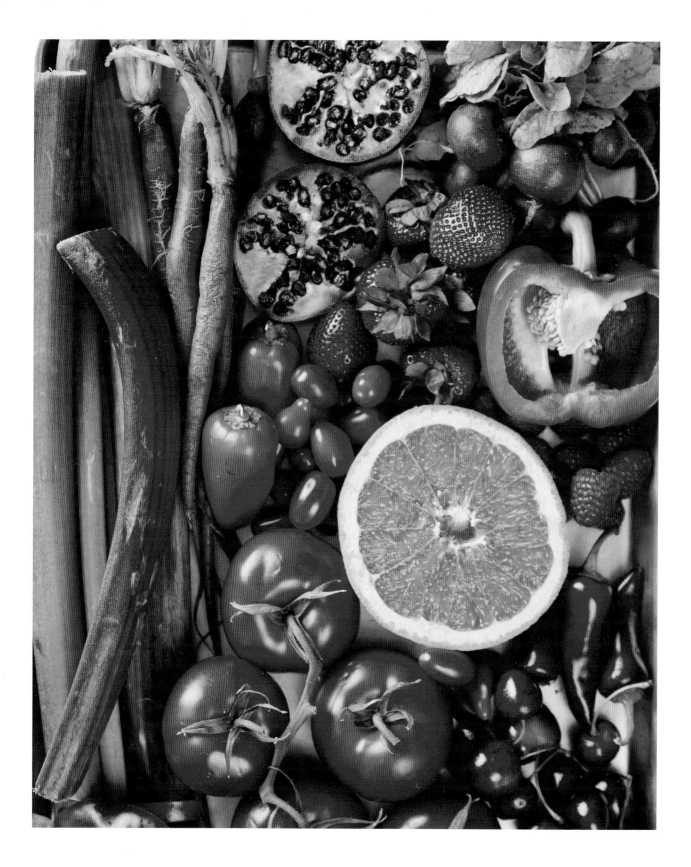

Salads

Heirloom Tomato Quinoa Salad

vegetarian · nut-free · gluten-free

Makes 4 servings

1 cup uncooked quinoa

2 cups water

2 tablespoons extra virgin olive oil

1 tablespoon fresh lemon juice

1 clove garlic, minced

½ teaspoon salt

2 cups assorted heirloom grape tomatoes (red, yellow and/or a combination), halved

¼ cup crumbled feta cheese

¼ cup chopped fresh basil

1. Place quinoa in fine-mesh strainer; rinse well under cold running water. Bring 2 cups water and quinoa to a boil in small saucepan. Reduce heat to low; cover and simmer 10 to 15 minutes or until quinoa is tender and water is absorbed.

2. Meanwhile, whisk oil, lemon juice, garlic and salt in large bowl until smooth and well blended. Gently stir in tomatoes and quinoa. Cover and refrigerate at least 30 minutes.

3. Top with cheese and basil just before serving.

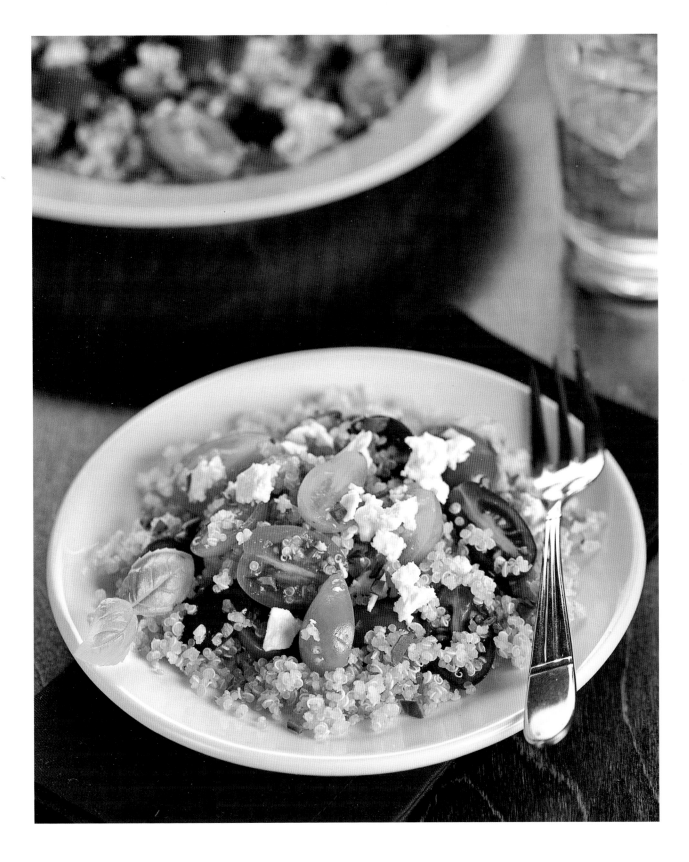

Southwestern Tuna Salad

dairy-free · **nut-free** · **gluten-free**

Makes 4 servings

---

12 ounces raw tuna steaks (about 1 inch thick)

2 limes, divided

2½ teaspoons canola oil, divided

1 pint cherry or grape tomatoes, halved

1 jalapeño pepper, seeded and minced

¼ cup diced ripe avocado

1 green onion, chopped

1 tablespoon chopped fresh cilantro

¼ teaspoon salt

¼ teaspoon ground cumin

⅛ teaspoon black pepper

Lime wedges (optional)

1. Place tuna steaks in shallow glass bowl. Juice one lime; pour over tuna. Marinate at room temperature 30 minutes, turning once.

2. Brush stovetop grill pan with 1 teaspoon oil; heat over medium heat 30 seconds. Add tuna steaks; cook 5 to 6 minutes per side or until cooked to desired degree of doneness. Remove and set aside until cooled to room temperature. Cut into bite-size chunks.

3. Place tomatoes, jalapeño, avocado, green onion and cilantro in large bowl. Add tuna.

4. Juice remaining lime; measure 4 teaspoons. Whisk remaining 1½ teaspoons oil, lime juice, salt, cumin and black pepper in small bowl. Pour over salad; toss to coat. Garnish with lime wedges, if desired.

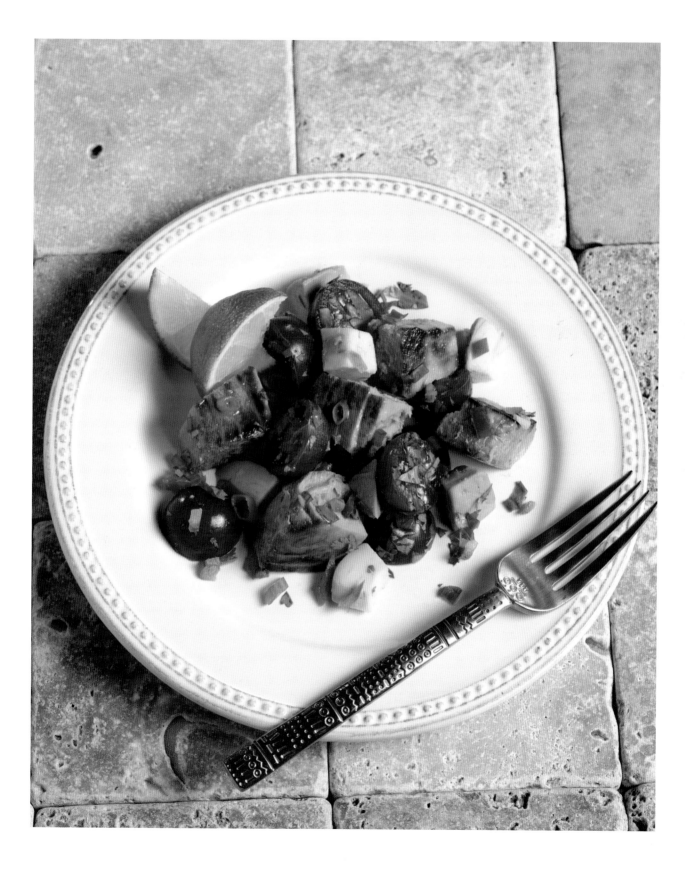

Bulgur, Tuna and Avocado Salad

dairy-free · **nut-free**

Makes 3 servings

⅔ **cup water**

⅓ **cup uncooked bulgur**

1 **cup halved grape tomatoes**

1 **can (5 ounces) tuna packed in water, drained and flaked**

¼ **cup finely chopped red onion**

1 **stalk celery, thinly sliced**

¼ **cup finely chopped avocado**

1 **tablespoon minced fresh Italian parsley**

1 **to 2 tablespoons fresh lemon juice**

4 **teaspoons chicken broth**

1 **teaspoon extra virgin olive oil**

½ **teaspoon salt**

⅛ **teaspoon black pepper**

1. Bring water to a boil in small saucepan. Stir in bulgur. Reduce heat to low. Cover and simmer 8 minutes or until bulgur swells and most of water is absorbed. Remove from heat; let stand, covered, 10 minutes.

2. Combine tomatoes, tuna, onion and celery in large bowl. Stir in bulgur, avocado and parsley.

3. Whisk lemon juice, broth, oil, salt and pepper in small bowl. Pour over salad; toss gently to mix. Refrigerate 2 hours before serving.

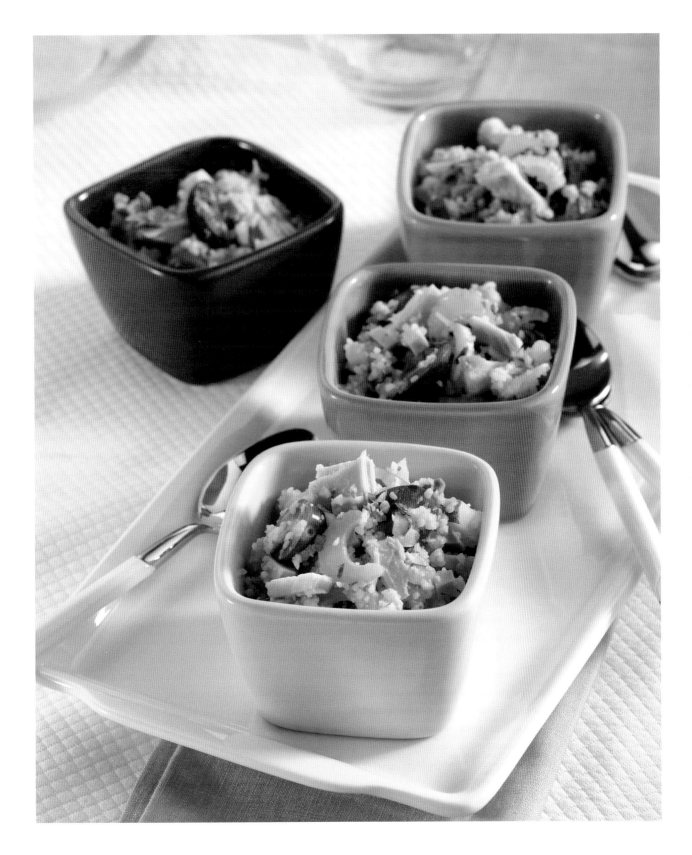

Zesty Zucchini-Chickpea Salad

vegetarian · nut-free · gluten-free

Makes 4 to 6 servings

- **3 medium zucchini (about 6 ounces each), halved lengthwise and cut into ¼-inch slices**
- **½ teaspoon salt**
- **5 tablespoons white wine vinegar**
- **1 clove garlic, minced**
- **¼ teaspoon dried thyme, crushed**
- **½ cup extra virgin olive oil**
- **1 cup cooked chickpeas**
- **½ cup sliced pitted black olives**
- **3 green onions, minced**
- **1 canned chipotle pepper in adobo sauce, minced**
- **1 ripe avocado, cut into ½-inch cubes**
- **⅓ cup crumbled feta cheese *or* 3 tablespoons grated Romano cheese**
- **1 head Boston lettuce, separated into leaves**
- **Sliced tomatoes**

1. Place zucchini in medium bowl; sprinkle with salt. Toss to mix. Spread zucchini on several layers of paper towels. Let stand at room temperature 30 minutes to drain.

2. Combine vinegar, garlic and thyme in large bowl. Gradually whisk in oil until blended.

3. Pat zucchini dry; add to dressing. Add chickpeas, olives and green onions; toss to coat. Cover and refrigerate at least 30 minutes or up to 4 hours, stirring occasionally.

4. Just before serving, stir in chipotle pepper; fold in avocado and feta. Place lettuce and tomatoes on serving plates; top with salad.

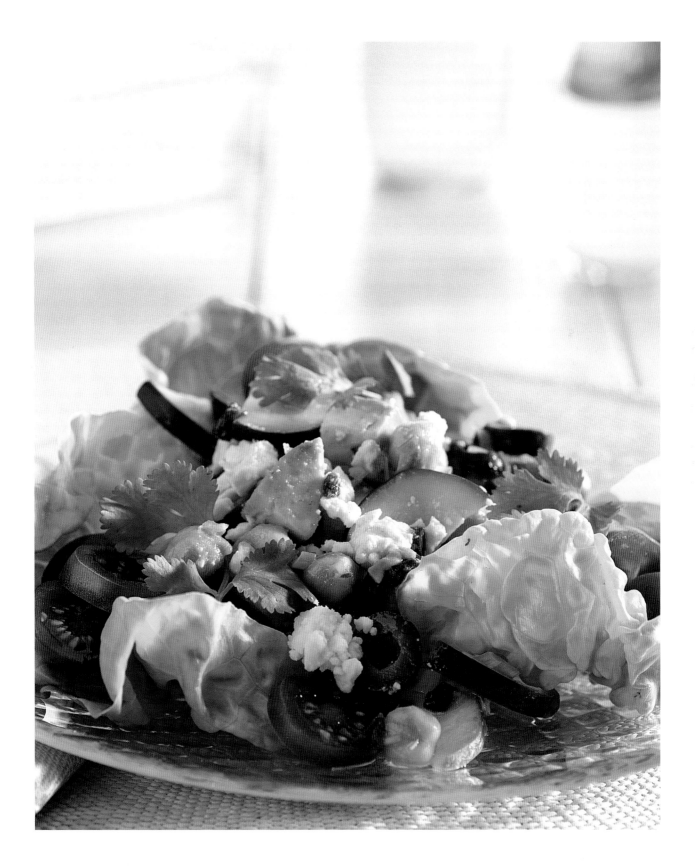

Fennel, Olive and Radicchio Salad

dairy-free · **nut-free** · **gluten-free**

Makes 4 servings

½ **cup Italian- or Greek-style black olives, divided**

¼ **cup extra virgin olive oil**

1 **tablespoon fresh lemon juice**

1 **flat anchovy fillet** *or* **½ teaspoon anchovy paste**

¼ **teaspoon salt**

Dash black pepper

1 **bulb fennel**

1 **head radicchio***

Fennel tops (optional)

*Or substitute 2 heads of Belgian endive.

1. For dressing, cut 3 olives in half; remove and discard pits. Place pitted olives, oil, lemon juice and anchovy in food processor; process 5 seconds. Add salt and pepper; process about 5 seconds or until olives are finely chopped. Set aside.

2. Cut off and discard fennel stalks, reserving green leafy tops for garnish. Cut off and discard root end of bulb and any discolored parts. Cut bulb lengthwise into 8 wedges; separate each wedge into segments.

3. Separate radicchio leaves; rinse thoroughly and drain well. Arrange radicchio leaves, fennel and remaining olives on serving plate. Spoon dressing over salad; garnish with fennel leaves. Serve immediately.

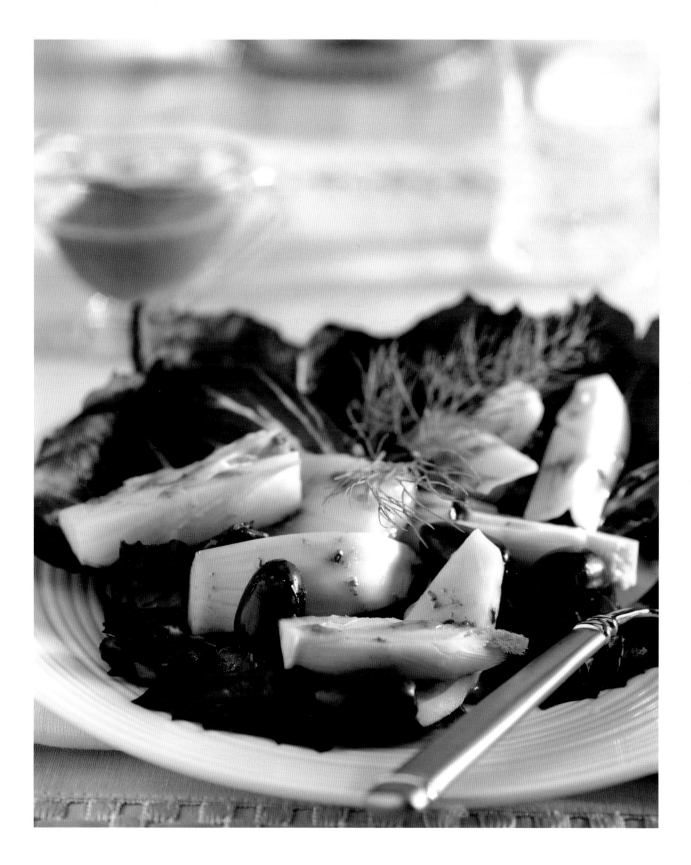

Warm Salmon Salad

dairy-free · nut-free · **gluten-free**

Makes 4 servings

Chive Vinaigrette (recipe
follows)

2 cups water

¼ cup chopped onion

2 tablespoons red wine
vinegar

¼ teaspoon black pepper

1¼ pounds small unpeeled red
potatoes

1 pound salmon steaks

6 cups torn washed mixed
salad greens

2 medium tomatoes, cut into
wedges

16 kalamata olives, sliced

1. Prepare Chive Vinaigrette.

2. Combine water, onion, vinegar and pepper
in large saucepan; bring to a boil over medium-
high heat. Add potatoes. Reduce heat; cover and
simmer 10 minutes or until fork-tender. Transfer
potatoes to cutting board with slotted spoon; cool
slightly. Return water to a boil.

3. Rinse salmon and pat dry with paper towels.
Add fish to water; simmer gently 4 to 5 minutes or
until fish is opaque and flakes easily when tested
with fork. *Do not boil.*

4. Cut potatoes into thick slices; place in medium
bowl. Add ⅓ cup Chive Vinaigrette; toss to coat.

5. Carefully transfer fish to cutting board. Let stand
5 minutes. Remove skin and bones from fish; cut
into 1-inch cubes.

6. Place salad greens on four plates. Arrange fish,
potatoes, tomatoes and olives on top. Drizzle with
remaining Chive Vinaigrette.

Chive Vinaigrette

vegan · vegetarian · dairy-free · nut-free · **gluten-free**

Makes about ⅔ cup

⅓ cup extra virgin olive oil

¼ cup red wine vinegar

2 tablespoons finely chopped
fresh chives

2 tablespoons finely chopped
fresh parsley

½ teaspoon salt

⅛ teaspoon white pepper

1. Combine oil, vinegar, chives, parsley, salt and
pepper in jar with tight-fitting lid; shake well to
combine.

2. Refrigerate until ready to use.

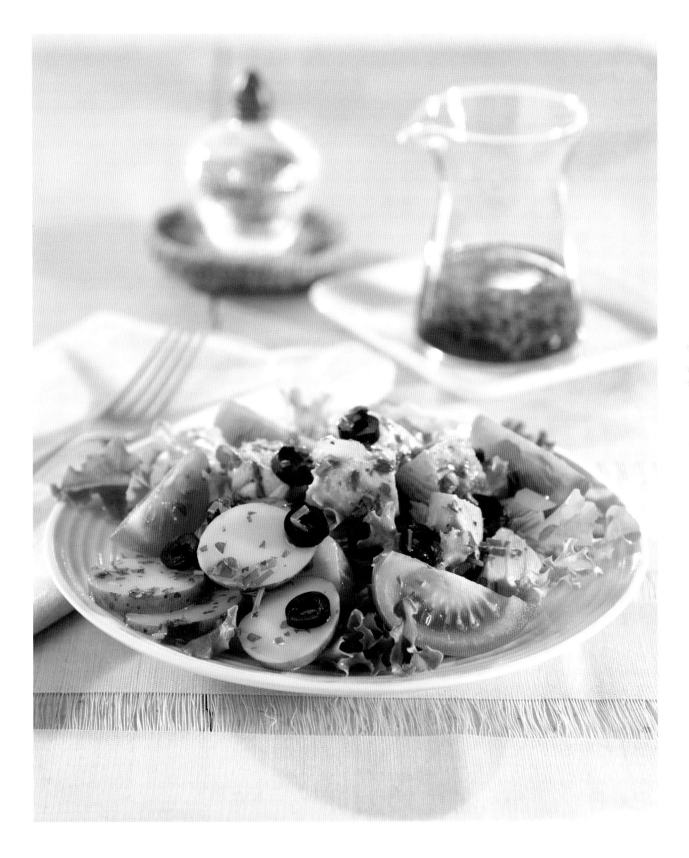

Spinach-Melon Salad

vegetarian · dairy-free · **nut-free** · **gluten-free**

Makes 6 servings

6 cups packed fresh spinach

4 cups mixed melon balls (cantaloupe, honeydew and/or watermelon)

1 cup zucchini ribbons*

½ cup sliced red bell pepper

¼ cup thinly sliced red onion

¼ cup red wine vinegar

2 tablespoons honey

2 teaspoons extra virgin olive oil

2 teaspoons fresh lime juice

1 teaspoon poppy seeds

1 teaspoon dried mint

To make ribbons, thinly slice zucchini lengthwise with vegetable peeler or spiral cutter.

1. Combine spinach, melon, zucchini, bell pepper and onion in large bowl.

2. Combine vinegar, honey, oil, lime juice, poppy seeds and mint in small jar with tight-fitting lid; shake well. Pour over salad; toss gently to coat.

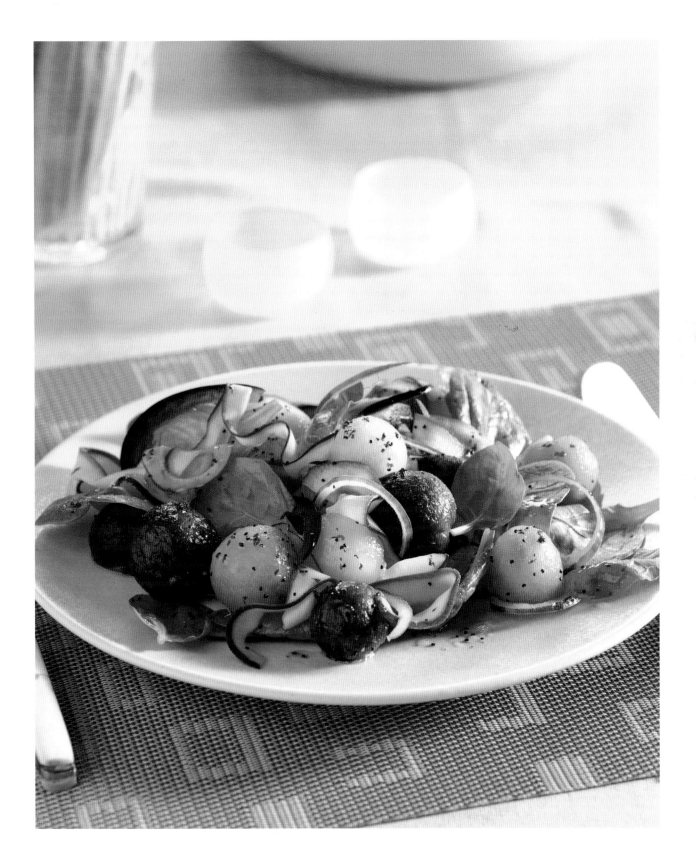

Shrimp and Spinach Salad

nut-free

Makes 6 servings

4	**cups packed baby spinach**
12	**ounces medium cooked shrimp, chilled**
1	**small red onion, thinly sliced**
1	**cup cooked whole wheat penne pasta or macaroni**
½	**cup plain Greek yogurt**
1	**tablespoon white wine vinegar**
1	**tablespoon extra virgin olive oil**
1	**clove garlic, minced**
¼	**teaspoon smoked paprika**
¼	**teaspoon dried oregano**
¼	**teaspoon black pepper**
⅛	**teaspoon salt**

1. Combine spinach, shrimp, onion and pasta in large bowl.

2. Whisk yogurt, vinegar, oil, garlic, paprika, oregano, pepper and salt in small bowl. Spoon over salad and toss to coat.

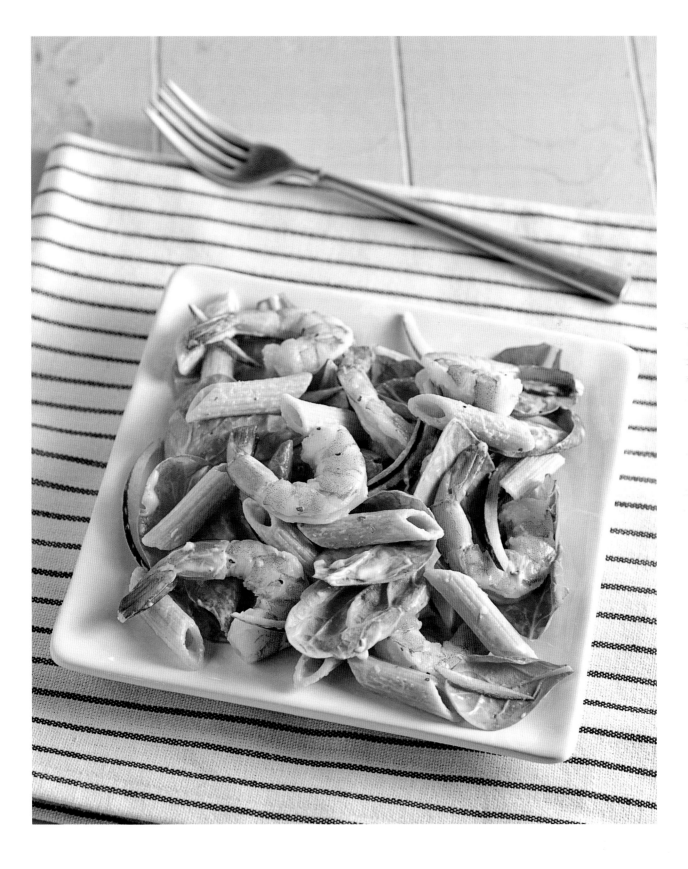

Tuna Tabbouleh Salad

dairy-free · **nut-free**

Makes 4 servings

1 cup water

¾ cup uncooked fine-grain bulgur wheat

3 tablespoons fresh lemon juice

1 teaspoon grated lemon peel

1 clove garlic, minced

½ teaspoon salt

⅛ teaspoon black pepper

1 tablespoon extra virgin olive oil

1 cup red or yellow cherry tomatoes, quartered

1 cup chopped cucumber

¼ cup finely chopped red onion

3 cans (5 ounces each) chunk white albacore tuna packed in water, drained and flaked

½ cup chopped fresh Italian parsley

4 cups watercress, tough stems removed

1. Bring water to a boil in small saucepan. Stir in bulgur. Remove from heat; cover and let stand 15 minutes. Place bulgur in fine-mesh strainer; run under cold water to cool.

2. Meanwhile, whisk lemon juice, lemon peel, garlic, salt and pepper in large bowl. Slowly whisk in oil. Add tomatoes, cucumber, onion and bulgur; stir to combine. Gently fold in tuna and parsley. Serve over watercress.

Tip: To make this dish gluten-free, replace bulgur wheat with 1 cup quinoa cooked according to package directions.

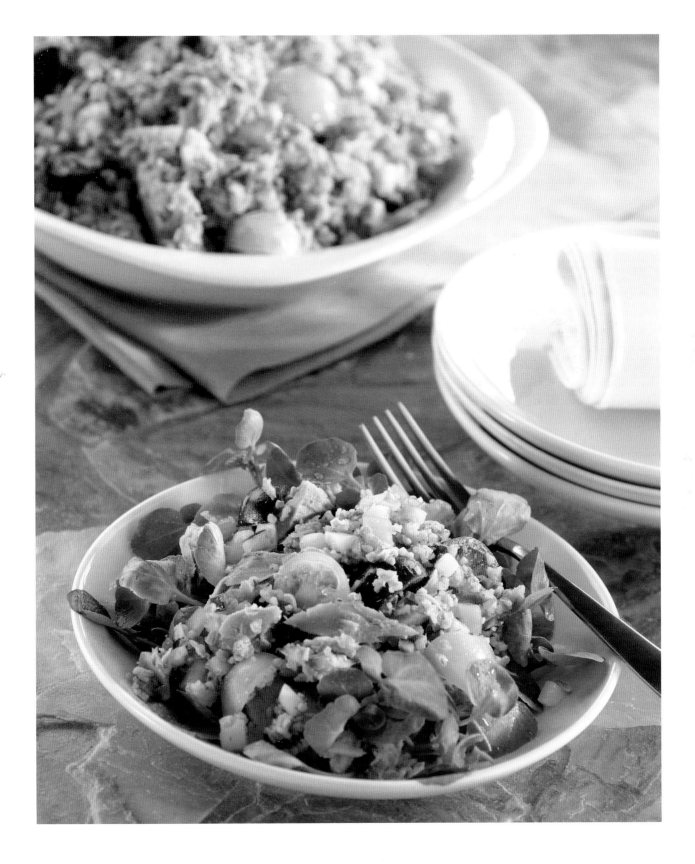

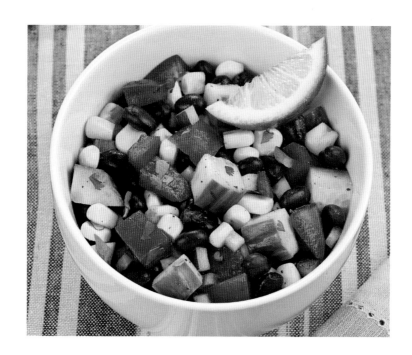

Southwest Gazpacho Salad

vegan · vegetarian · dairy-free · nut-free · gluten-free

Makes 2 servings

1 **cup cooked black beans**

1 **cup diced tomato**

⅔ **cup corn**

½ **cup diced cucumber**

2 **tablespoons diced red onion**

1 **tablespoon finely chopped fresh cilantro**

3 **tablespoons tomato juice**

1 **tablespoon fresh lime juice**

2 **teaspoons extra virgin olive oil**

½ **teaspoon chili powder**

¼ **teaspoon salt**

Pinch black pepper

1. Combine beans, tomato, corn, cucumber, onion and cilantro in large bowl.

2. Whisk tomato juice, lime juice, oil, chili powder, salt and pepper in small bowl. Pour over salad; mix gently.

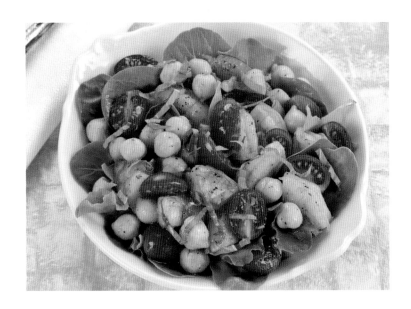

Mediterranean Shrimp and Bean Salad

dairy-free · **nut-free** · **gluten-free**

Makes 4 servings

10 **ounces large cooked shrimp, cut into bite-size pieces**

1½ **cups grape or cherry tomatoes, halved**

1 **large shallot, minced**

¾ **cup cooked chickpeas**

¼ **cup shredded fresh basil**

¼ **teaspoon salt**

¼ **teaspoon paprika**

¼ **teaspoon black pepper**

⅛ **teaspoon dried oregano**

3 **tablespoons tomato or vegetable juice**

1 **tablespoon white wine vinegar**

1 **tablespoon extra virgin olive oil**

1. Combine shrimp, tomatoes, shallot, chickpeas and basil in large bowl.

2. Combine salt, paprika, pepper and oregano in small bowl. Gradually whisk in tomato juice. Whisk in vinegar and oil. Pour over salad; toss gently to coat.

Green Salad with Pears and Pecans

vegetarian · **gluten-free**

Makes 4 servings

½ **cup Greek yogurt**

1 **tablespoon finely minced onion**

1 **tablespoon extra virgin olive oil**

1 **tablespoon balsamic vinegar**

¼ **teaspoon salt**

⅛ **teaspoon black pepper**

1 **bag (10 ounces) mixed salad greens**

2 **ripe pears, cored and thinly sliced**

½ **cup pecans, toasted***

¼ **cup pomegranate seeds**

¼ **cup finely shredded Parmesan cheese (optional)**

*To toast pecans, spread in single layer in heavy skillet. Cook over medium heat 1 to 2 minutes or until nuts are lightly browned, stirring frequently. Remove from skillet. Cool completely.

1. Whisk yogurt, onion, oil, vinegar, salt and pepper in small bowl until well blended.

2. Arrange greens evenly on four plates. Top with pears, pecans and pomegranate seeds. Drizzle with dressing and sprinkle with cheese, if desired.

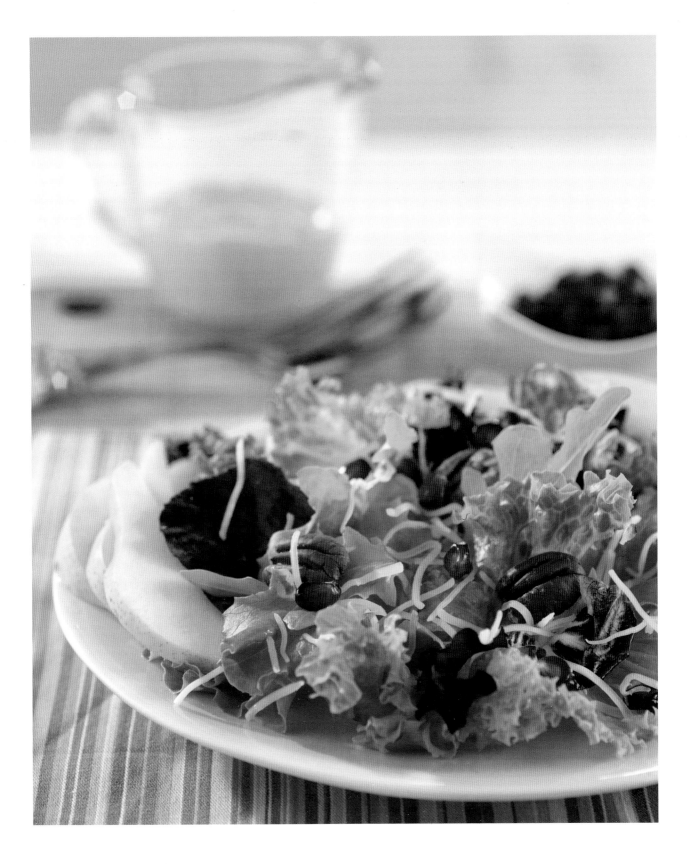

Spinach Salad with Pomegranate Vinaigrette

vegetarian · gluten-free

Makes 4 servings

1 package (5 ounces) baby spinach

½ cup pomegranate seeds

¼ cup crumbled goat cheese

2 tablespoons chopped walnuts, toasted*

¼ cup pomegranate juice

2 tablespoons extra virgin olive oil

1 tablespoon honey

1 tablespoon red wine vinegar

¼ teaspoon salt

¼ teaspoon black pepper

To toast walnuts, spread in single layer in heavy skillet. Cook over medium heat 1 to 2 minutes or until nuts are lightly browned, stirring frequently. Remove from skillet. Cool completely.

1. Combine spinach, pomegranate seeds, goat cheese and walnuts in large bowl.

2. Whisk pomegranate juice, oil, honey, vinegar, salt and pepper in small bowl until well blended. Pour over salad; gently toss to coat. Serve immediately.

Tip: For easier removal of pomegranate seeds, cut a pomegranate into pieces and immerse in a bowl of cold water. The membrane that holds the seeds in place will float to the top; discard it and collect the seeds. Containers of ready-to-use pomegranate seeds are available in the refrigerated produce section of well-stocked supermarkets.

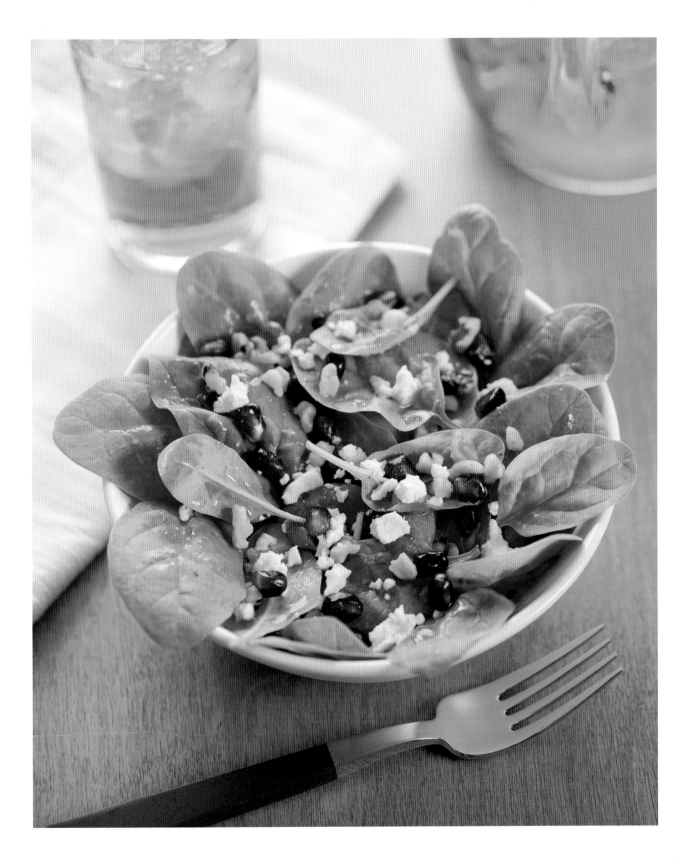

Greek Salad with Dairy-Free "Feta"

vegan · vegetarian · dairy-free · nut-free · **gluten-free**

Makes 4 to 6 servings

Dairy-Free "Feta"

- 1 **package (14 ounces) firm or extra firm tofu**
- ½ **cup extra virgin olive oil**
- ¼ **cup fresh lemon juice**
- 2 **teaspoons salt**
- 2 **teaspoons dried Greek or Italian seasoning**
- ½ **teaspoon black pepper**
- 1 **teaspoon onion powder**
- ½ **teaspoon garlic powder**

Salad

- 1 **pint grape tomatoes, halved**
- 2 **seedless cucumbers, quartered lengthwise and sliced**
- 1 **yellow bell pepper, slivered**
- 1 **small red onion, thinly sliced**

1. For "feta," cut tofu crosswise into two pieces, each about 1 inch thick. Place on cutting board lined with paper towels; top with layer of paper towels. Place weighted baking dish on top of tofu. Let stand 30 minutes to drain. Pat tofu dry and crumble into large bowl.

2. Combine oil, lemon juice, salt, Greek seasoning and black pepper in small jar with tight-fitting lid; shake until well blended. Reserve ¼ cup mixture for salad dressing. Add onion powder and garlic powder to remaining mixture; pour over tofu and stir to coat. Cover and refrigerate 2 hours or overnight.

3. For salad, combine tomatoes, cucumbers, bell pepper and onion in serving bowl. Add tofu and reserved dressing; toss gently.

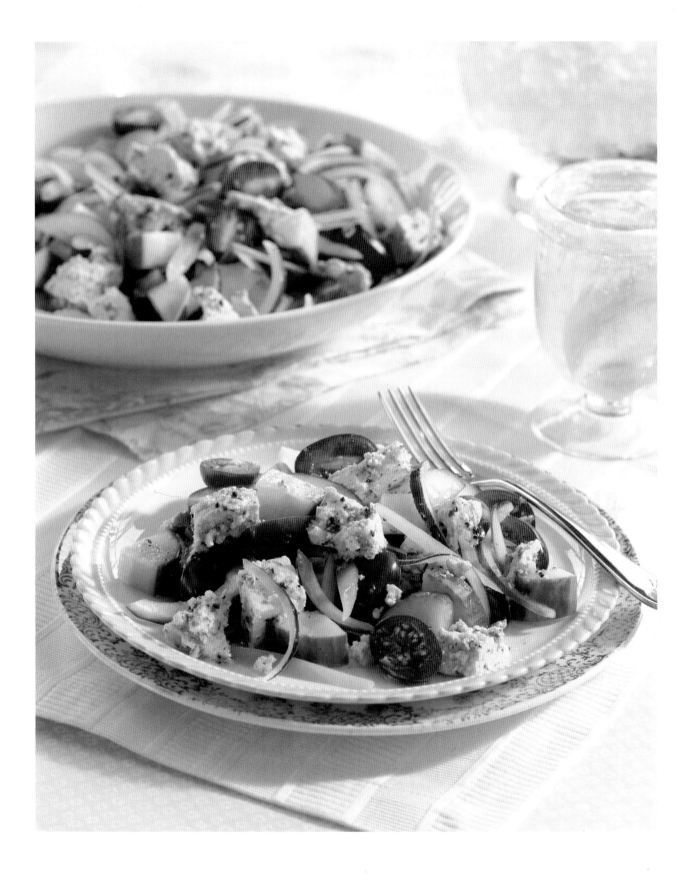

Broiled Chicken Salad

dairy-free · **nut-free** · **gluten-free**

Makes 4 servings

Basil Vinaigrette (recipe follows) or Chive Vinaigrette (page 66)

4 **boneless skinless chicken breasts (about 4 ounces each)**

1 **can (about 15 ounces) black beans, rinsed and drained**

2 **green onions, chopped**

2 **cups cooked corn**

2 **tablespoons chopped pimiento**

2 **tablespoons chopped fresh cilantro**

2 **large tomatoes, cut into wedges**

1. Prepare Basil Vinaigrette; set aside.

2. Preheat broiler. Position rack about 4 inches from heat source. Broil chicken 8 minutes or until browned on both sides and no longer pink in center, turning once halfway through cooking.

3. Meanwhile, combine beans, green onions and 1 tablespoon dressing in medium bowl. Combine corn, pimiento and chopped cilantro in another medium bowl.

4. Slice chicken diagonally; arrange on salad plates. Serve with tomato wedges, bean mixture, corn mixture and remaining dressing.

Basil Vinaigrette

vegan · **vegetarian** · dairy-free · **nut-free** · **gluten-free**

Makes about ½ cup

---

6 **tablespoons extra virgin olive oil**

2 **tablespoons balsamic vinegar**

2 **tablespoons minced fresh basil**

1 **clove garlic, minced**

1 **teaspoon minced fresh chives**

½ **teaspoon salt**

¼ **teaspoon black pepper**

Combine all ingredients in small bowl; whisk until blended.

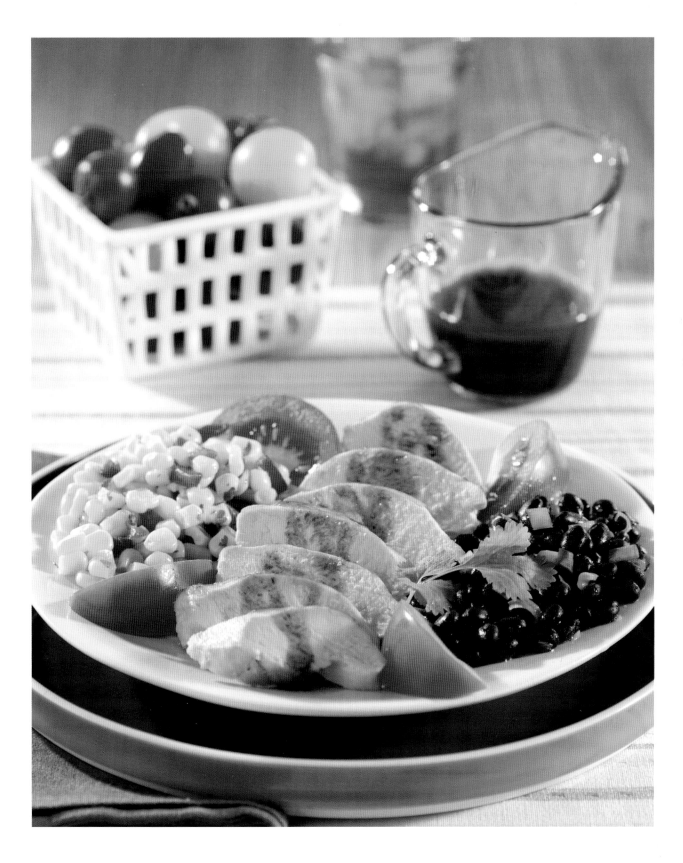

Grapefruit Salad with Raspberry Dressing

vegetarian · dairy-free · **nut-free** · **gluten-free**

Makes 4 servings

2 cups washed watercress

2 cups mixed salad greens

3 medium grapefruit, peeled, sectioned and seeded

8 ounces jicama, cut into thin strips

1 cup fresh raspberries

2 tablespoons chopped green onion

1 tablespoon honey

1 teaspoon balsamic vinegar

½ teaspoon dry mustard

1. Combine watercress and salad greens in large bowl; divide evenly among four plates. Top with grapefruit and jicama.

2. Reserve 12 raspberries for garnish. Combine remaining raspberries, green onion, honey, vinegar and mustard in food processor or blender; process until smooth and well blended.

3. Drizzle dressing over salads; garnish with reserved raspberries. Serve immediately.

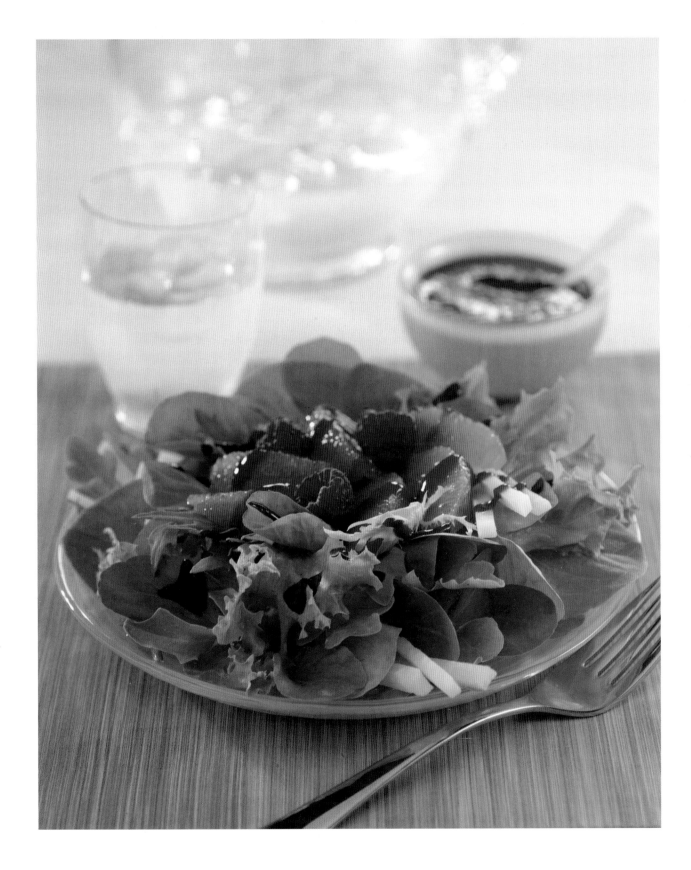

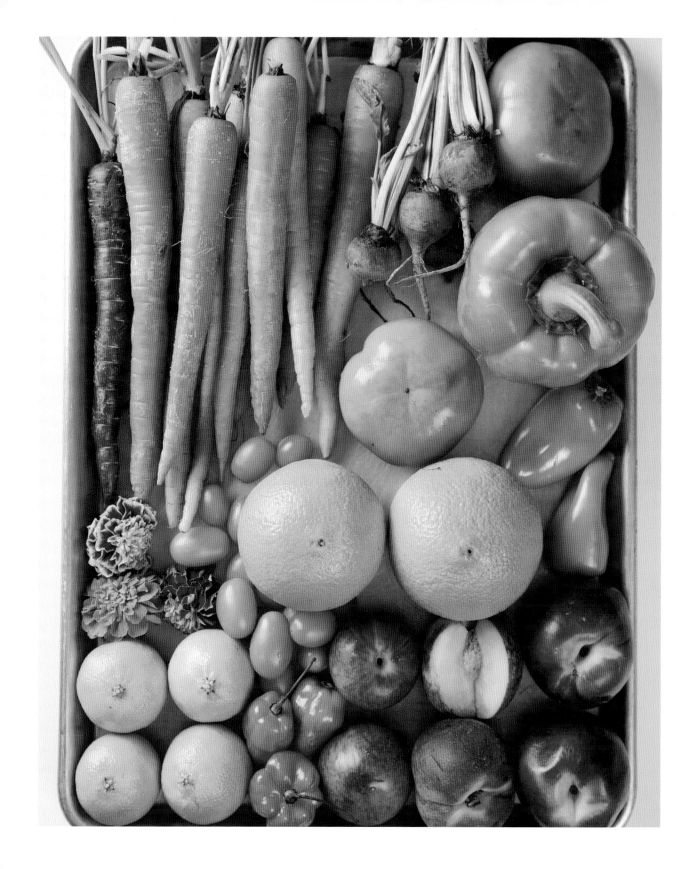

Soups

Butternut Squash and Millet Soup

dairy-free · **nut-free** · **gluten-free**

Makes 6 servings

1 red bell pepper

1 teaspoon canola oil

2¼ cups diced butternut squash

1 red onion, chopped

1 teaspoon curry powder

½ teaspoon smoked paprika

½ teaspoon salt

⅛ teaspoon black pepper

2 cups chicken broth

2 boneless skinless chicken breasts (about 4 ounces each), cooked and chopped

1 cup cooked millet

1. Preheat broiler. Place bell pepper on rack in broiler pan 3 to 5 inches from heat source or hold over open gas flame on long-handled metal fork. Turn bell pepper often until blistered and charred on all sides. Transfer to resealable food storage bag; seal bag and let stand 15 to 20 minutes to loosen skin. Remove loosened skin with paring knife. Cut off top and scrape out seeds; discard. Coarsely chop bell pepper.

2. Heat oil in large saucepan over high heat. Add squash, bell pepper and onion; cook and stir 5 minutes. Add curry powder, paprika, salt and black pepper. Pour in broth; bring to a boil. Cover and cook 7 to 10 minutes or until vegetables are tender.

3. Purée soup in saucepan with immersion blender or in batches in food processor or blender. Return soup to saucepan. Stir in chicken and millet; cook until heated through.

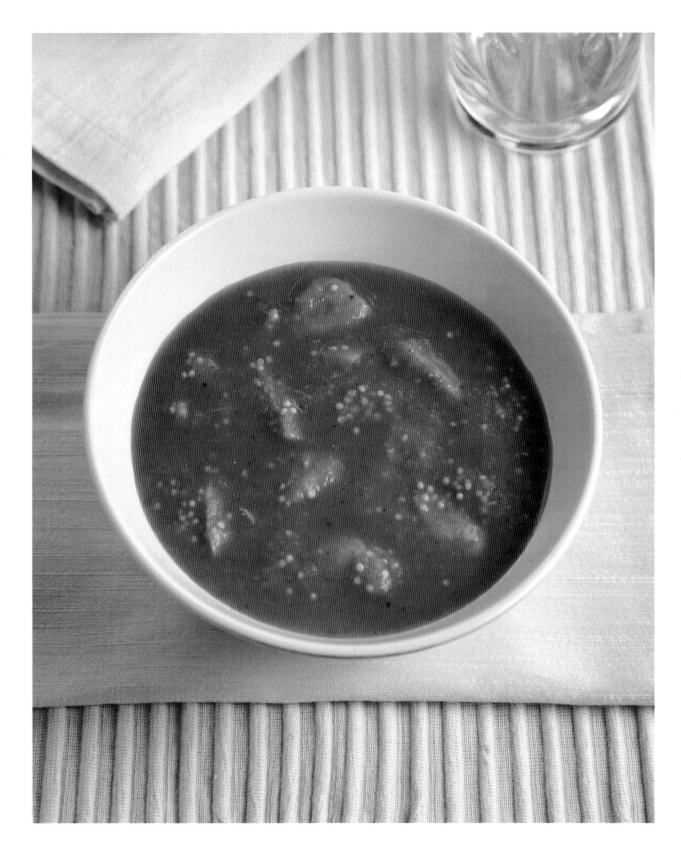

Chilled Fresh Tomato Basil Soup

vegan · vegetarian · dairy-free · nut-free · gluten-free

Makes 4 servings

- 3 **medium tomatoes, seeded and diced**
- 1 **cup finely chopped green bell pepper**
- ½ **medium cucumber, peeled, seeded and finely chopped**
- ¼ **cup chopped fresh basil**
- ¼ **cup finely chopped peperoncini**
- 1 **cup water**
- 3 **tablespoons red wine vinegar**
- 2 **tablespoons extra virgin olive oil**
- ½ **teaspoon salt**
- 2 **tablespoons chopped fresh parsley**

1. Combine tomatoes, bell pepper, cucumber, basil and peperoncini in large bowl.

2. Whisk water, vinegar and salt in small bowl. Stir in parsley. Pour over vegetables; stir to coat.

3. Combine and refrigerate 30 minutes to allow flavors to blend.

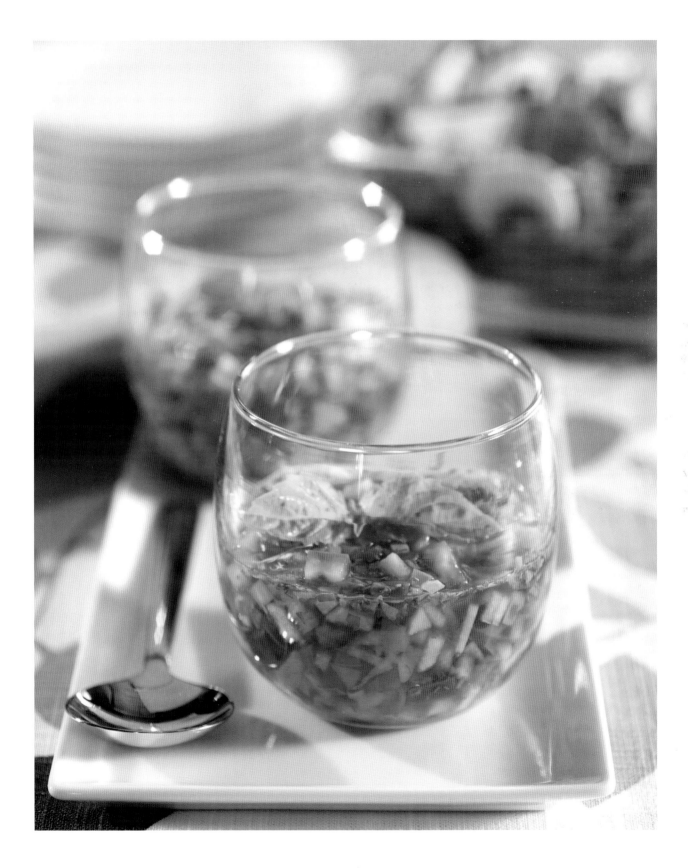

French Lentil Soup

vegan · vegetarian · dairy-free · nut-free · gluten-free

Makes 4 to 6 servings

3 tablespoons extra virgin olive oil

1 medium onion, chopped

1 carrot, chopped

1 stalk celery, chopped

1 clove garlic, minced

3 to 4 cups vegetable broth

1 can (about 14 ounces) stewed tomatoes

8 ounces dried lentils, rinsed and sorted

   Salt and black pepper

1. Heat oil in large skillet over medium heat. Add onion, carrot, celery and garlic; cook and stir 9 to 10 minutes or until vegetables are tender but not browned.

2. Add 3 cups broth, tomatoes and lentils; bring to a boil over high heat. Reduce heat; cover and simmer 30 minutes or until lentils are tender, adding additional 1 cup broth if needed. Season to taste with salt and pepper.

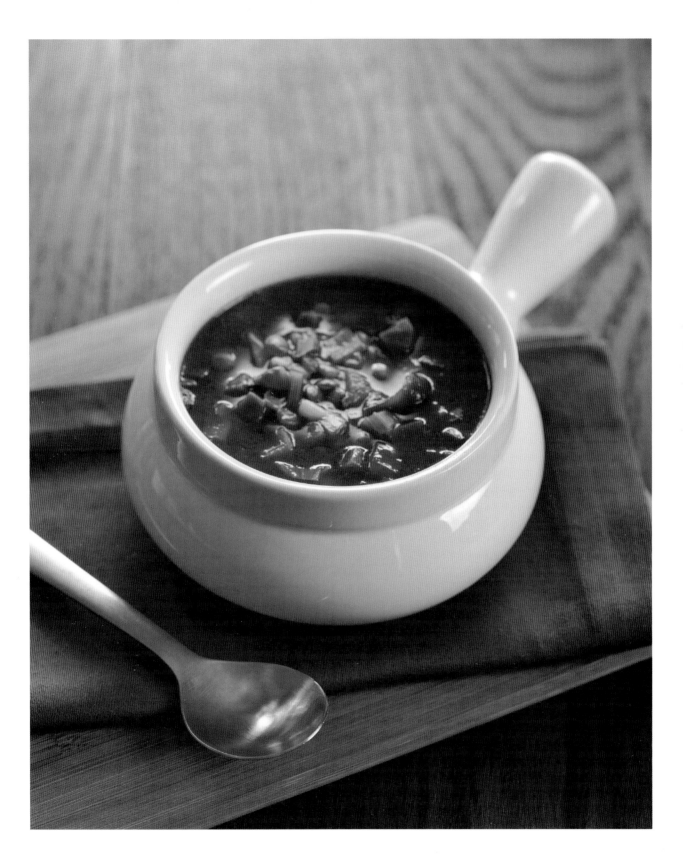

Sweet Potato Minestrone

vegetarian · nut-free · gluten-free

Makes 4 servings

1 tablespoon extra virgin
   olive oil

¾ cup diced onion

½ cup diced celery

3 cups water

2 cups diced peeled sweet
   potatoes

1 can (about 15 ounces) Great
   Northern beans, rinsed
   and drained

1 can (about 14 ounces)
   diced tomatoes

¾ teaspoon dried rosemary

½ teaspoon salt

⅛ teaspoon black pepper

2 cups coarsely chopped kale
   leaves (lightly packed)

4 tablespoons freshly
   grated Parmesan cheese
   (optional)

1. Heat oil in large saucepan or Dutch oven over medium-high heat. Add onion and celery; cook and stir 4 minutes or until onion is softened.

2. Stir in water, sweet potatoes, beans, tomatoes, rosemary, salt and pepper. Bring to a boil. Reduce heat; cover and simmer 30 minutes. Add kale; cover and cook 10 minutes or until kale and sweet potatoes are tender.

3. Ladle soup into bowls; sprinkle with cheese, if desired.

Note: Choose kale in small bunches with firm leaves and a rich, deep color. Avoid bunches with limp, wilted or discolored leaves. To remove the tough stems, make a V-shaped cut where the stem joins the leaf. Stack the leaves and cut them into pieces.

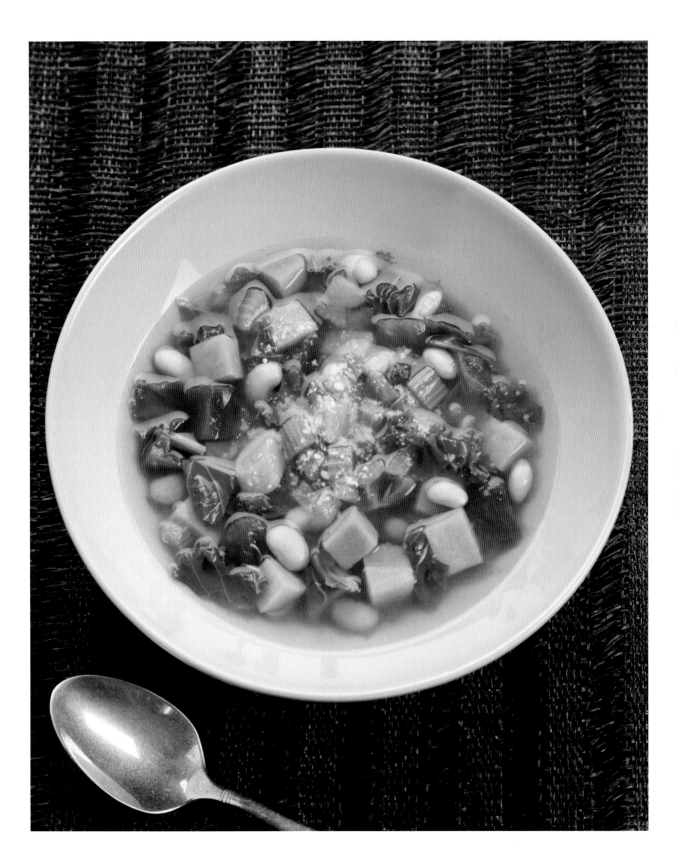

Red Bell Pepper Soup

vegan · **vegetarian** · dairy-free · **nut-free** · **gluten-free**

Makes 4 to 6 servings

2 tablespoons extra virgin olive oil

8 red bell peppers, stemmed, seeded and quartered

1 onion, thinly sliced

3 cloves garlic, minced

1 teaspoon dried oregano

1 teaspoon black pepper

2 tablespoons balsamic vinegar

1½ tablespoons fresh thyme leaves *or* 4 to 6 fresh thyme sprigs (optional)

1. Coat slow cooker with oil. Add bell peppers, onion, garlic, oregano and black pepper; gently mix. Cover; cook on HIGH 4 hours or until bell peppers are very tender; stirring halfway through cooking.

2. Purée soup in slow cooker using immersion blender or transfer in batches to blender or food processor and blend until smooth. Stir in vinegar. Ladle soup into bowls; garnish with thyme.

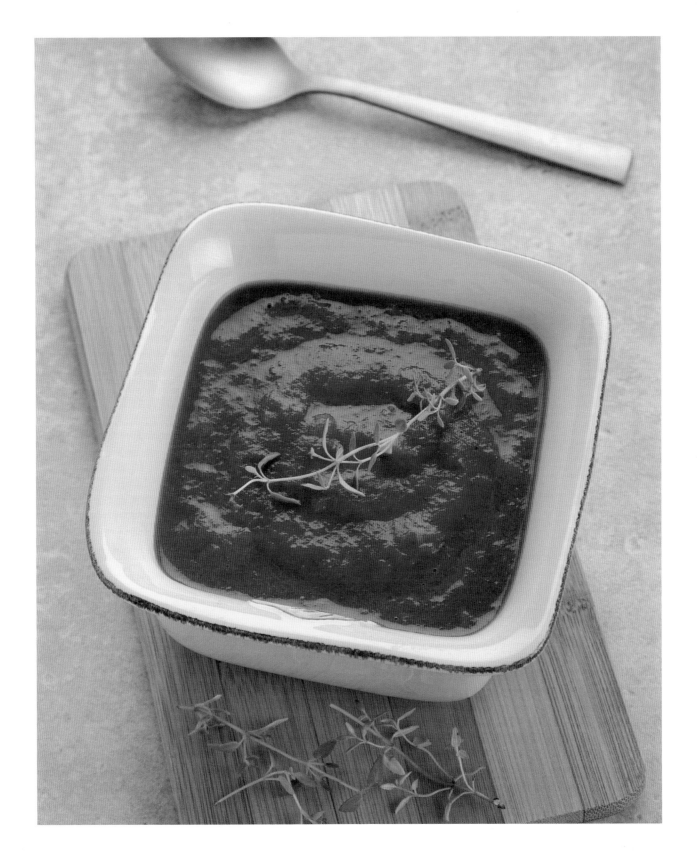

Coconut Curry Chicken Soup

nut-free · gluten-free

Makes 4 servings

- 3 **cups chicken broth**
- 8 **boneless skinless chicken thighs**
- 1 **cup chopped onion, divided**
- 1 **teaspoon salt, divided**
- 4 **whole cloves**
- 1 **tablespoon coconut oil**
- 2 **tablespoons curry powder**
- 1¼ **cups coconut milk**
- ¼ **cup plus 1 tablespoon chopped fresh mint, divided**
- 3 **tablespoons crystallized ginger**
- ¼ **teaspoon ground cloves**
- 1½ **cups half-and-half**
- 3 **cups cooked rice**
  Lime wedges (optional)

1. Bring broth to a boil in large skillet over high heat. Add chicken, ½ cup onion, ½ teaspoon salt and whole cloves. Return to a boil. Reduce heat; cover and simmer 40 minutes or until chicken is very tender. Remove chicken; set aside. Strain cooking liquid; reserve 1 cup.

2. Melt coconut oil in same skillet over medium-high heat. Add remaining ½ cup onion; cook and stir 4 minutes or until onion is translucent. Sprinkle curry powder over onions; cook 20 seconds or just until fragrant, stirring constantly.

3. Add coconut milk, 1 tablespoon mint, ginger, ground cloves and reserved cooking liquid to skillet. Cover and simmer 10 minutes. Add chicken; cover and simmer 15 minutes. Stir in half-and-half and remaining ½ teaspoon salt. Shred chicken slightly. Cook 1 minute or until heated through. Sprinkle with remaining ¼ cup mint. Spoon rice over each serving and garnish with lime wedges.

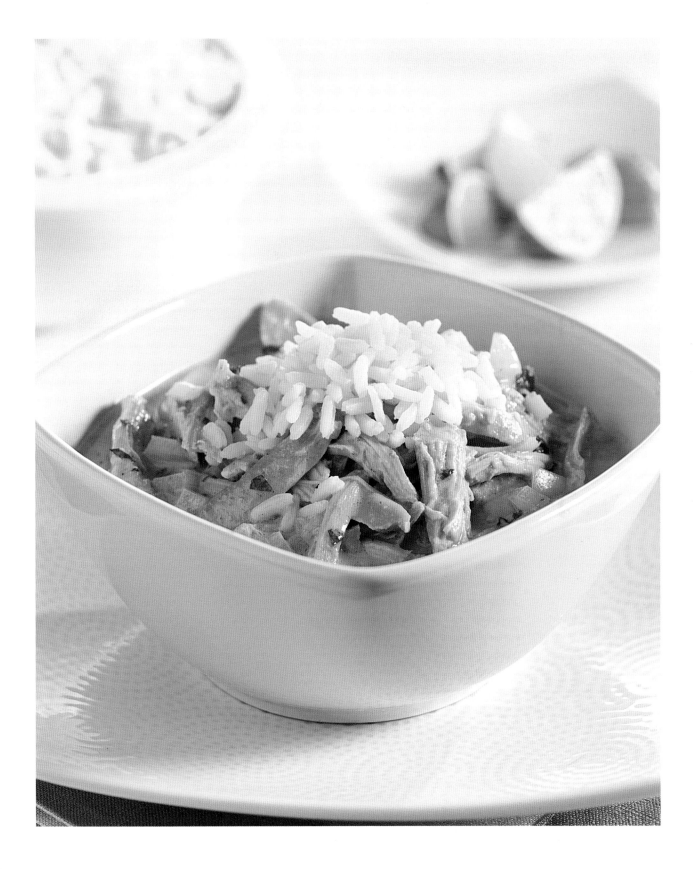

Lentil Vegetable Stew

vegan · vegetarian · dairy-free · nut-free · gluten-free

Makes 8 servings

3 tablespoons canola oil

1 large onion, coarsely chopped

1 can (28 ounces) crushed tomatoes

2 cups water

1 tablespoon curry powder

1 tablespoon cider vinegar

1½ teaspoons salt

1½ teaspoons ground cumin

1½ teaspoons ground coriander

1 teaspoon ground ginger

1¼ cups dried lentils, rinsed

2 cups cauliflower florets

1 cup chopped red bell pepper

1 cup chopped yellow squash

1. Heat oil in large saucepan over medium heat. Add onion; cook and stir 5 minutes or until softened. Stir in tomatoes, water, curry powder, vinegar, salt, cumin, coriander and ginger. Stir in lentils; bring to a boil. Reduce heat to medium-low; simmer 35 to 40 minutes or until lentils begin to soften.

2. Add cauliflower, bell pepper and squash; cook 30 to 40 minutes or until vegetables and lentils are tender.

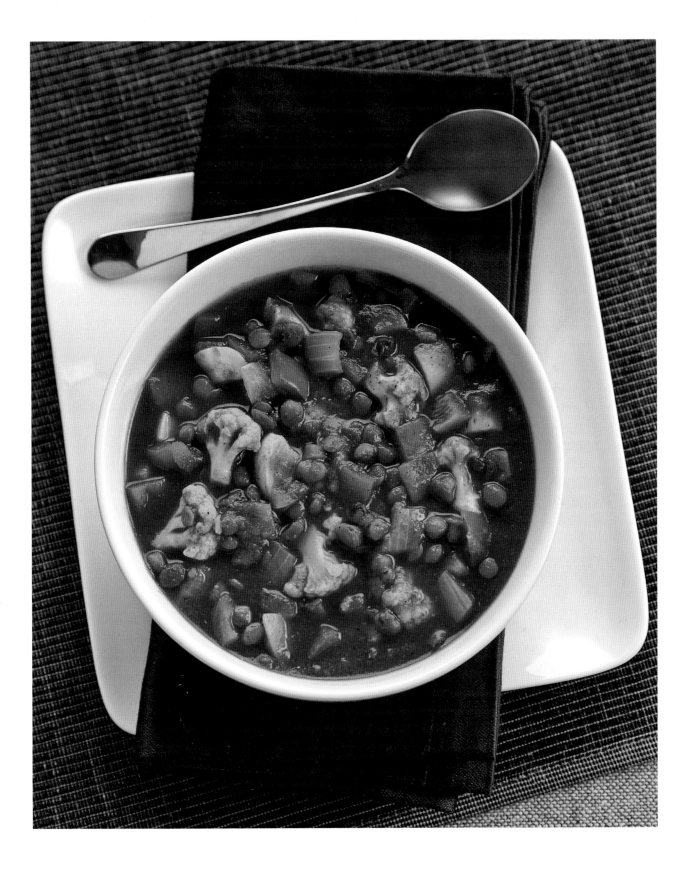

Albondigas Soup

dairy-free · **nut-free** · **gluten-free**

Makes 6 servings

6 cups chicken broth

1 onion, chopped

¼ cup sliced celery

1 pound lean ground beef

2 eggs, lightly beaten

¼ cup blue or yellow cornmeal

1 clove garlic, minced

1 tablespoon chopped fresh mint *or* 1 teaspoon dried mint

½ teaspoon salt

¼ teaspoon ground cumin

Dash black pepper

1 carrot, chopped

1 zucchini, chopped

1 yellow squash, chopped

½ bunch spinach, stemmed and sliced ½ inch thick

2 limes, cut into wedges

1. Combine broth, onion and celery in large saucepan or Dutch oven; bring to a boil over high heat. Reduce heat to medium-low; simmer 10 minutes.

2. Meanwhile, combine beef, eggs, cornmeal, garlic, mint, salt, cumin and pepper in medium bowl. Shape mixture into 1-inch balls.

3. Add meatballs to broth mixture; simmer 5 minutes. Skim off fat and foam from surface of broth. Add carrot, zucchini and squash; simmer 20 minutes or until vegetables are tender.

4. Add spinach; simmer 5 minutes. Serve with lime wedges.

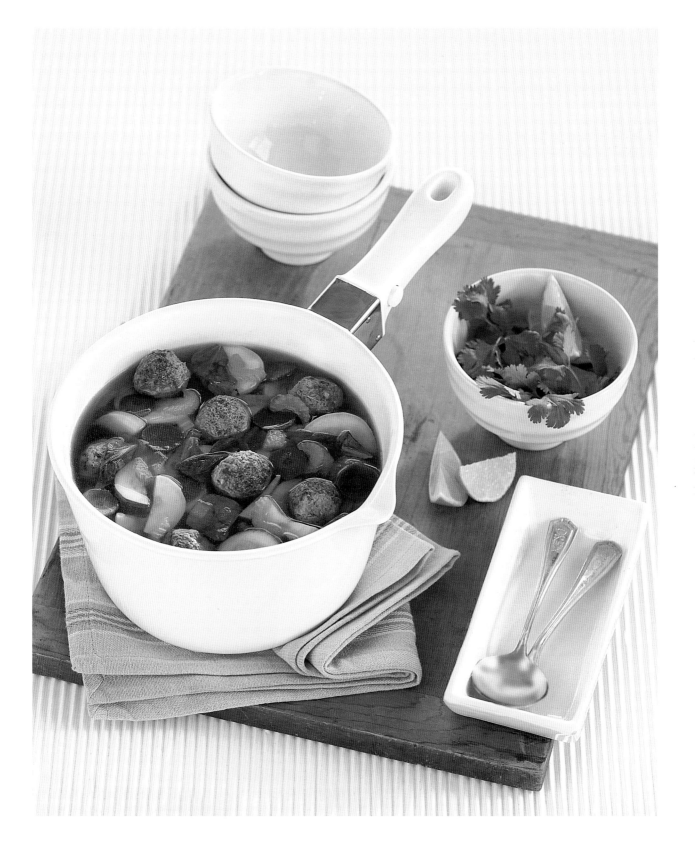

Salmon and Wild Rice Chowder

nut-free

Makes 8 servings

1 teaspoon coconut oil

1 red onion, chopped

1 red bell pepper, chopped

1 cup green beans, cut into 1-inch pieces

1½ teaspoons minced fresh dill

1 teaspoon salt

⅛ teaspoon black pepper

3 cups vegetable broth

1 cup cooked wild rice

12 ounces skinless salmon fillet, cut into 1-inch pieces

½ cup milk

2 teaspoons all-purpose flour

1. Melt coconut oil in large saucepan over high heat. Add onion, bell pepper and green beans; cook and stir 5 minutes. Stir in dill, salt and black pepper. Pour in broth; bring to a simmer.

2. Add wild rice and salmon. Reduce heat to low; cover and simmer 6 to 8 minutes or until salmon flakes easily when tested with fork.

3. Whisk milk into flour in small bowl until smooth. Stir into saucepan. Cook until heated through.

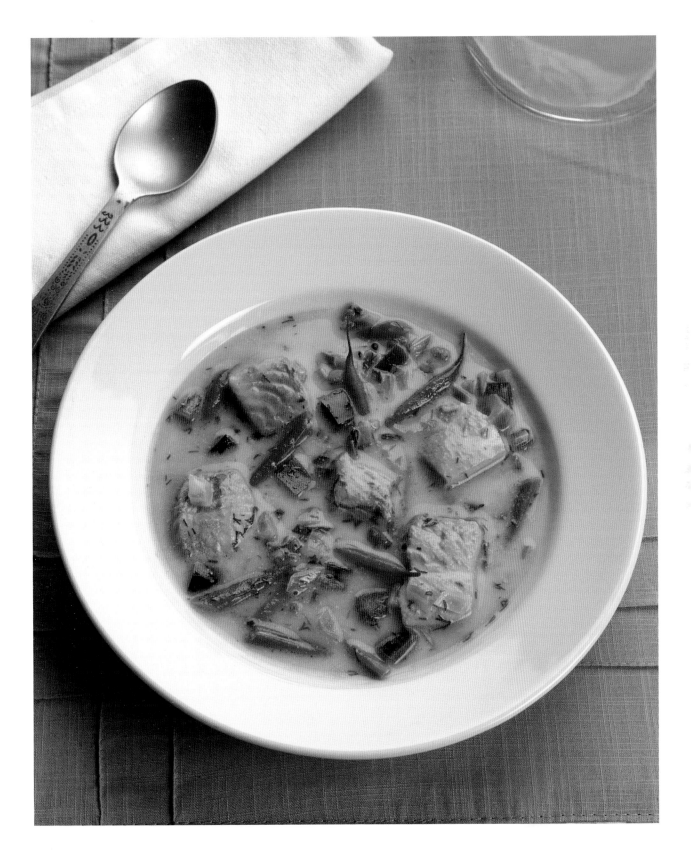

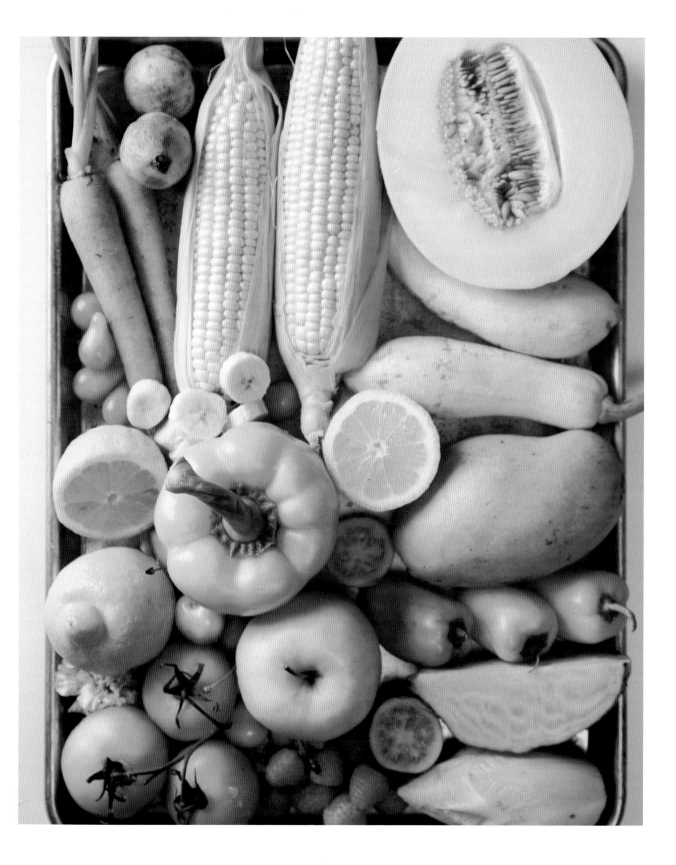

Entrées

Beef and Pepper Kabobs

dairy-free · **nut-free** · **gluten-free**

Makes 4 servings

8 ounces sirloin steak, trimmed of fat

2 teaspoons tamari

2 teaspoons red wine vinegar

1½ teaspoons Dijon mustard

1 teaspoon extra virgin olive oil

1 clove garlic, minced

⅛ teaspoon black pepper

1 tablespoon chicken or vegetable broth

2 bell peppers (any color)

4 green onions, trimmed

1. Slice steak into 16 strips, each about ¼ inch thick. Place in glass bowl. Whisk tamari, vinegar, mustard, oil, garlic and black pepper in small bowl until blended. Pour half of mixture over beef; stir broth into remaining mixture and refrigerate. Cover beef; marinate in refrigerator 2 to 3 hours, stirring occasionally.

2. Prepare grill for direct cooking.

3. Core and seed bell peppers; cut each into 12 chunks. Thread onto four metal skewers. Grill 5 to 7 minutes per side, or until well browned and tender, brushing once with marinade mixture. Grill green onions 3 to 5 minutes or until well browned, brushing once with marinade mixture. Coarsely chop green onions.

4. Thread beef strips onto four metal skewers. Grill 4 minutes, turning once and brushing occasionally with marinade. Serve beef with bell peppers and green onions.

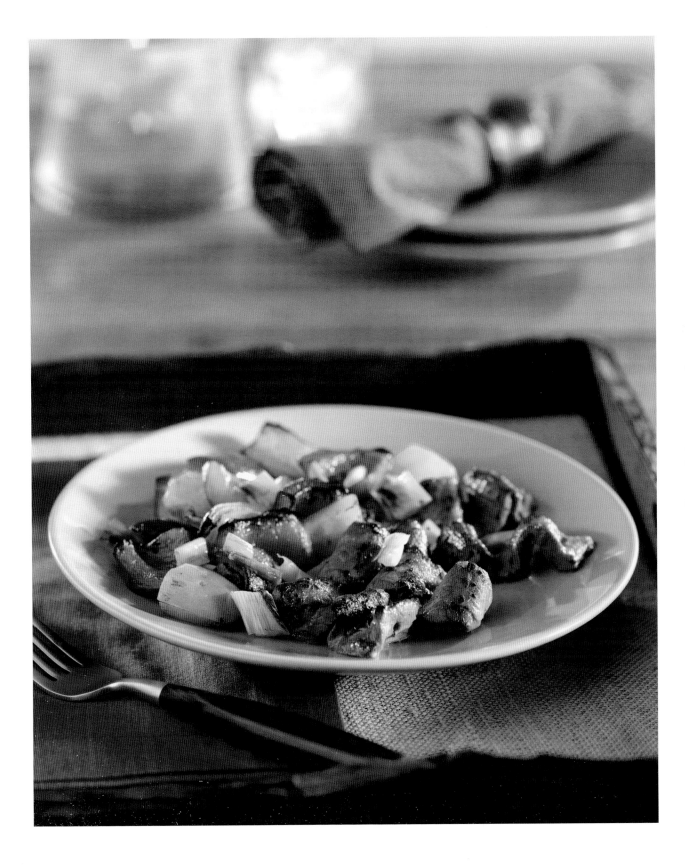

Farro Risotto with Mushrooms and Spinach

vegetarian · nut-free

Makes 4 servings

2 tablespoons extra virgin olive oil, divided

1 onion, chopped

12 ounces cremini mushrooms, stems trimmed and quartered

¾ teaspoon salt

¼ teaspoon black pepper

2 cloves garlic, minced

1 cup uncooked farro

1 sprig fresh thyme

4 cups vegetable broth

8 ounces baby spinach

½ cup grated Parmesan cheese

1. Heat 1 tablespoon oil in large skillet over medium heat. Add onion; cook 8 minutes or until tender. Transfer to slow cooker.

2. Add remaining 1 tablespoon oil to same skillet; heat over medium-high heat. Add mushrooms, salt and pepper; cook 6 to 8 minutes or until mushrooms have released their liquid and are browned, stirring occasionally. Add garlic; cook 1 minute. Stir in farro and thyme; cook 1 minute. Transfer to slow cooker.

3. Stir broth into slow cooker. Cover; cook on HIGH 3½ hours until farro is tender and broth is absorbed. Remove thyme sprig. Stir in spinach and cheese just before serving.

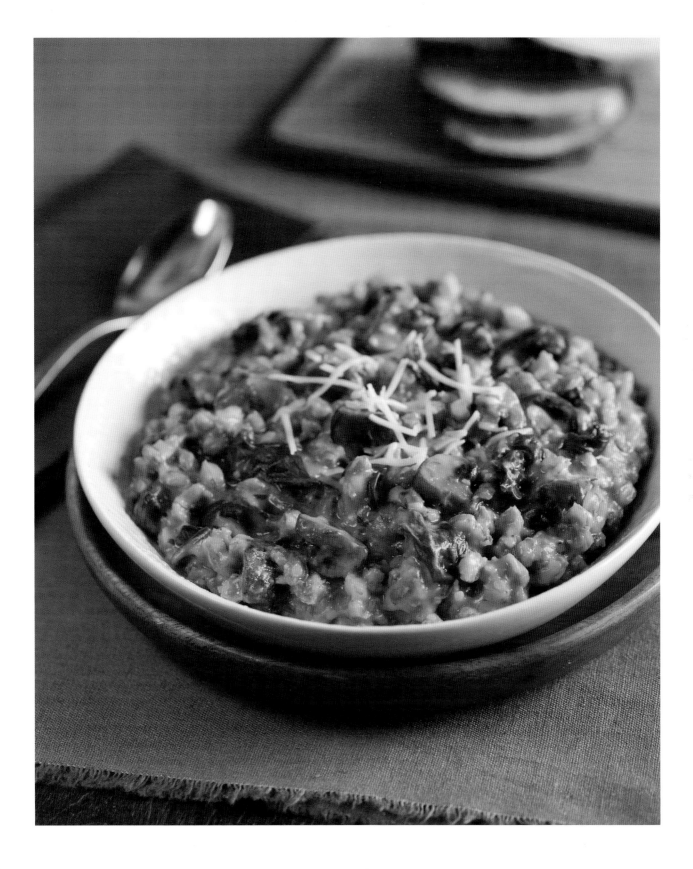

Greek Roast Chicken

dairy-free · **nut-free** · **gluten-free**

Makes 8 servings

1 whole chicken (4 to 5 pounds)

3 tablespoons extra virgin olive oil, divided

2 tablespoons chopped fresh rosemary leaves, plus whole sprigs

2 cloves garlic, minced

1 lemon

1¼ teaspoons salt, divided

½ teaspoon black pepper, divided

1 can (about 14 ounces) chicken broth, divided

2 sweet potatoes, peeled and cut into thick wedges

1 red onion, cut into ¼-inch wedges

1 pound fresh asparagus spears, trimmed

1. Preheat oven to 425°F. Place chicken in shallow roasting pan.

2. Combine 2 tablespoons oil, chopped rosemary and garlic in small bowl; brush over chicken.

3. Grate 1 teaspoon peel from lemon; set aside. Cut lemon into quarters; squeeze juice over chicken and place rinds and rosemary sprigs in chicken cavity. Sprinkle ¾ teaspoon salt and ¼ teaspoon pepper over chicken. Pour 1 cup broth into bottom of roasting pan; roast 30 minutes.

4. *Reduce oven temperature to 375°F.* Arrange sweet potatoes and onion wedges in single layer around chicken in roasting pan. Drizzle remaining broth and 1 tablespoon oil over vegetables; roast 15 minutes.

5. Arrange asparagus spears in roasting pan. Sprinkle remaining ½ teaspoon salt and ¼ teaspoon pepper over vegetables. Roast 10 minutes or until chicken is cooked through (165°F) and vegetables are tender. Transfer chicken to carving board. Tent with foil; let stand 10 to 15 minutes.

6. Sprinkle reserved lemon peel over chicken. Carve chicken and serve with vegetables and pan juices.

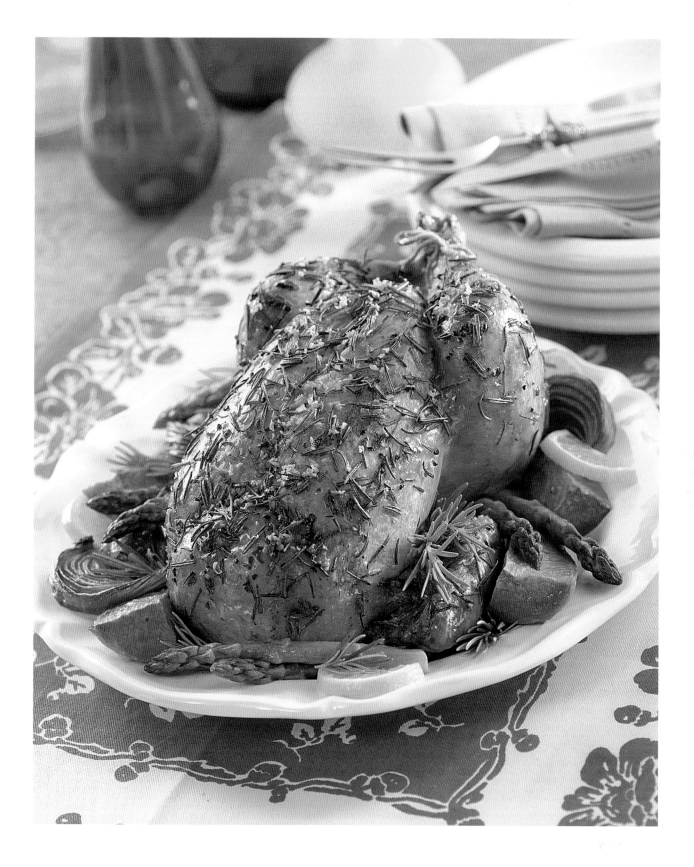

City Market Chicken Tarragon Penne

nut-free · gluten-free

Makes 4 servings

4 ounces uncooked gluten-free penne pasta

4 ounces fresh asparagus spears, trimmed and cut into 2-inch pieces

1½ cups diced cooked chicken breast

½ cup diced red onion

2 tablespoons canola oil

1 tablespoon chopped fresh tarragon

1 tablespoon fresh lemon juice

2 to 3 teaspoons coarse grain Dijon mustard

½ teaspoon salt

¼ teaspoon black pepper

2 ounces blue cheese, crumbled

1. Cook pasta according to package directions, adding asparagus during last 3 minutes of cooking.

2. Combine chicken, onion, oil, tarragon, lemon juice, mustard, salt and pepper in large bowl.

3. Drain pasta and asparagus; stir into chicken mixture. Add cheese; stir gently.

Tip: This dish is also good served cold. Stir in fresh lemon juice just before serving.

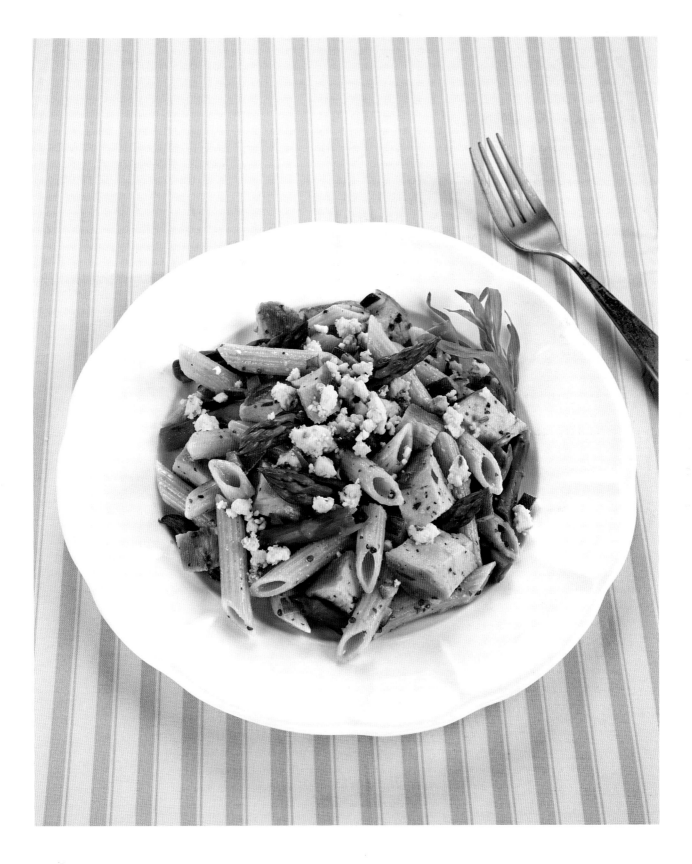

Spaghetti Squash with Tomato Sauce

dairy-free · **nut-free** · **gluten-free**

Makes 4 servings

1 spaghetti squash (about 4 pounds)

1 tablespoon extra virgin olive oil

2 cups sliced cremini mushrooms

½ cup diced onion

½ cup diced green bell pepper

1 can (about 14 ounces) diced tomatoes

½ cup tomato sauce

⅓ cup water

½ teaspoon dried oregano

¼ teaspoon salt

⅛ teaspoon black pepper

4 cooked chicken sausage links (3 ounces each), cut into pieces

2 tablespoons chopped fresh Italian parsley

1. Cut spaghetti squash lengthwise in half. Remove seeds. Place squash in 12×8-inch microwavable dish; cover with vented plastic wrap. Microwave on HIGH 9 minutes or until squash separates easily into strands when scraped with fork. Shred squash into large bowl with fork.

2. Heat oil in large skillet over medium-high heat. Add mushrooms, onion and bell pepper; cook and stir 7 minutes or until vegetables are tender.

3. Stir tomatoes, tomato sauce, water, oregano, salt and black pepper into skillet. Bring to a simmer. Reduce heat; cover and simmer 5 minutes. Stir in sausage pieces.

4. Divide squash evenly among four plates. Spoon sauce over squash; sprinkle with parsley.

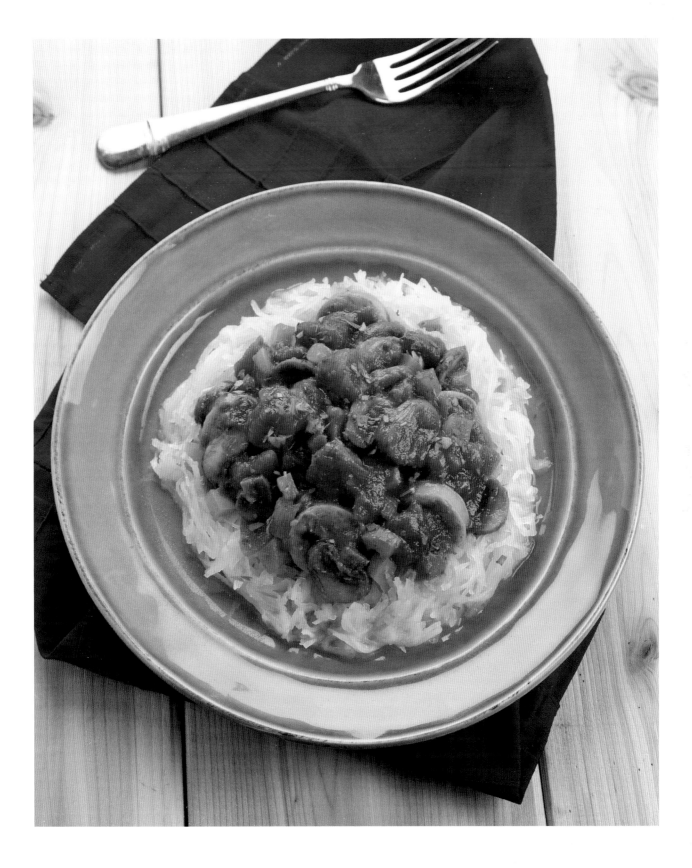

Soba Stir-Fry

vegan · **vegetarian** · dairy-free · **nut-free** · **gluten-free**

Makes 4 servings

8 ounces uncooked gluten-free soba (buckwheat) noodles

1 tablespoon extra virgin olive oil

2 cups sliced shiitake mushrooms

1 red bell pepper, cut into thin strips

2 whole dried red chiles *or* ¼ teaspoon red pepper flakes

1 clove garlic, minced

2 cups shredded napa cabbage

½ cup vegetable broth

2 tablespoons tamari

1 tablespoon rice wine or dry sherry

2 teaspoons cornstarch

1 package (14 ounces) firm tofu, drained and cut into 1-inch cubes

2 green onions, thinly sliced

1. Cook noodles according to package directions. Drain and set aside.

2. Heat oil in wok or large nonstick skillet over medium-high heat. Add mushrooms, bell pepper, dried chiles and garlic. Stir-fry 3 minutes or until mushrooms are tender. Add cabbage. Cover and cook 2 minutes or until cabbage is wilted.

3. Whisk broth, tamari and rice wine into cornstarch in small bowl until smooth. Stir sauce into vegetable mixture. Cook 2 minutes or until sauce is thickened.

4. Stir in tofu and noodles; toss gently until heated through. Sprinkle with green onions. Serve immediately.

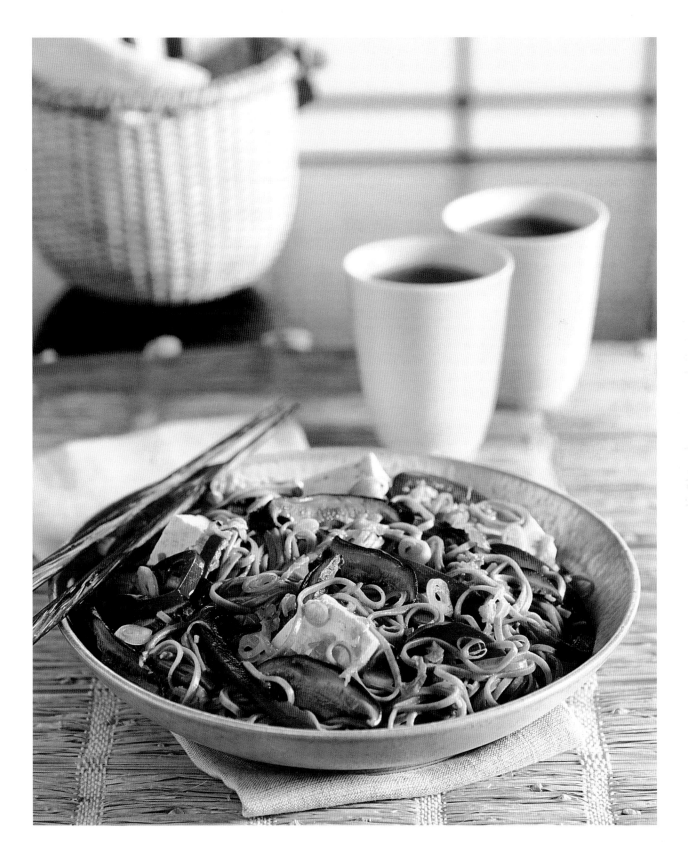

Quinoa Burrito Bowls

vegetarian · nut-free · gluten-free

Makes 4 servings

1 cup uncooked quinoa

2 cups water

2 tablespoons fresh lime juice, divided

¼ cup Greek yogurt

2 teaspoons canola oil

1 small onion, diced

1 red bell pepper, diced

1 clove garlic, minced

½ cup cooked black beans

½ cup corn

Shredded lettuce

Lime wedges (optional)

1. Place quinoa in fine-mesh strainer; rinse well under cold running water. Bring 2 cups water and quinoa to a boil in small saucepan. Reduce heat to low; cover and simmer 10 to 15 minutes or until quinoa is tender and water is absorbed. Stir in 1 tablespoon lime juice. Cover and keep warm.

2. Combine yogurt and remaining 1 tablespoon lime juice in small bowl; set aside.

3. Meanwhile, heat oil in large skillet over medium heat. Add onion and bell pepper; cook and stir 5 minutes or until softened. Add garlic; cook 1 minute. Add black beans and corn; cook 3 to 5 minutes or until heated through.

4. Divide quinoa among four serving bowls; top with black bean mixture, lettuce and sour cream mixture. Garnish with lime wedges.

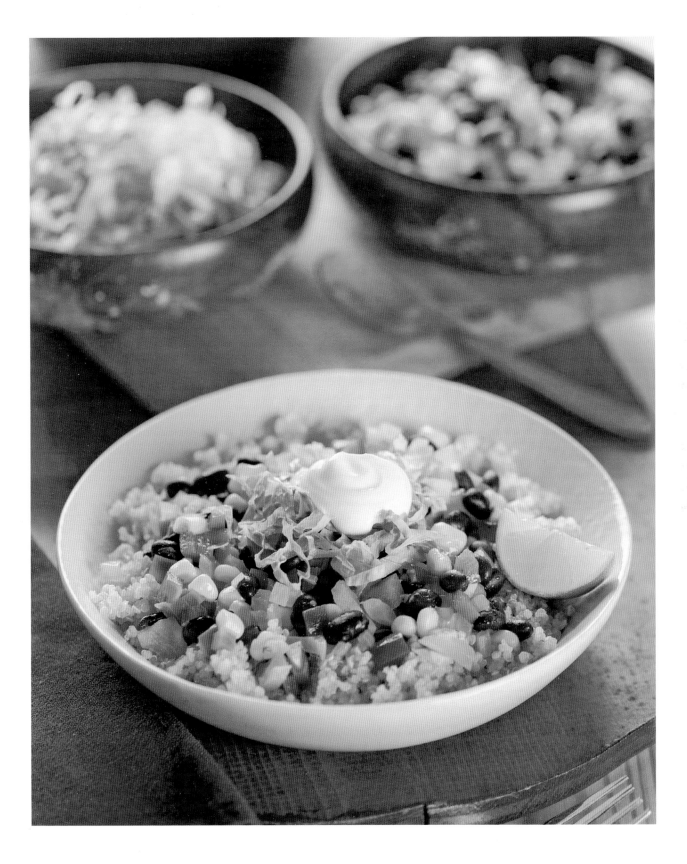

Spicy Tuna Sushi Bowl

nut-free · gluten-free

Makes 2 servings

- **2 tablespoons plain yogurt**
- **1 teaspoon sriracha or hot chile sauce**
- **3 teaspoons unseasoned rice wine vinegar, divided**
- **1 tuna steak (about 6 ounces)**
- **1 cup hot cooked brown rice**
- **½ cup diced cucumber**
- **½ ripe avocado, sliced**
- **Black sesame seeds**

1. Whisk yogurt, sriracha sauce and 1 teaspoon vinegar in small bowl. Rub half of sauce evenly over tuna. Marinate 10 minutes.

2. Meanwhile, stir remaining 2 teaspoons vinegar into rice; set aside.

3. Heat small nonstick skillet over medium-high heat. Cook tuna 2 minutes per side for medium-rare or until desired doneness is reached. Slice tuna.

4. Divide rice between two bowls. Top with cucumber, avocado and tuna slices. Sprinkle evenly with sesame seeds. Serve with remaining sauce.

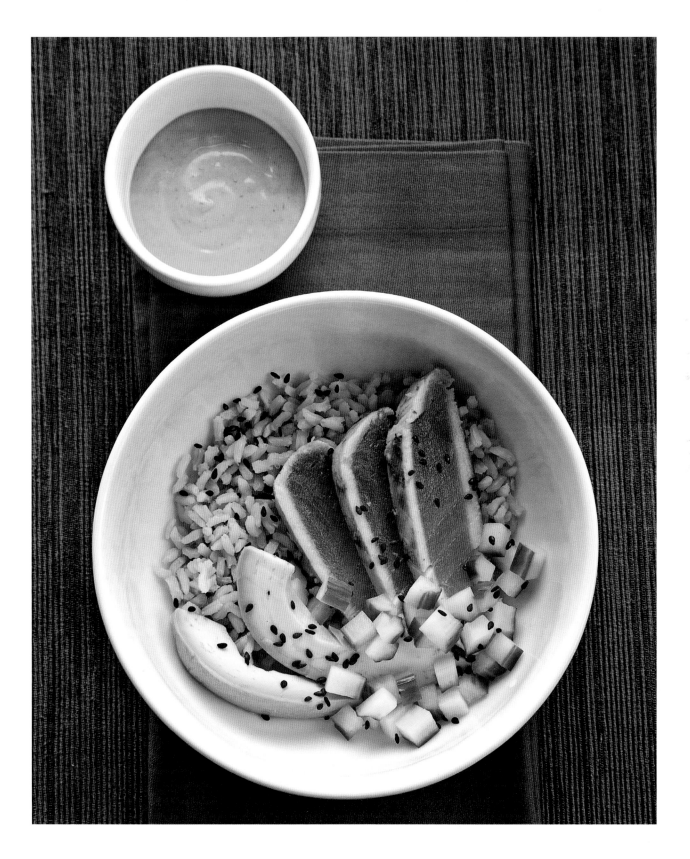

Roasted Beet Risotto

vegetarian · nut-free · gluten-free

Makes 4 servings

2 medium beets, trimmed

4 cups vegetable broth, divided

1 tablespoon canola oil

1 leek, finely chopped

1 cup uncooked arborio rice

½ cup crumbled goat cheese, plus additional for garnish

1 teaspoon dried Italian seasoning

¼ teaspoon salt

Juice of 1 lemon

Lemon wedges (optional)

1. Preheat oven to 400°F. Wrap each beet tightly in foil. Place on baking sheet. Roast 45 minutes to 1 hour or until knife inserted into centers goes in easily. Unwrap beets; let stand 15 minutes or until cool enough to handle. Peel beets and cut into bite-size pieces. Set aside.

2. Bring broth to a simmer in small saucepan; keep warm.

3. Heat oil in medium saucepan over medium-high heat. Add leek; cook and stir 1 to 2 minutes or until softened. Add rice; cook and stir 1 to 2 minutes or until rice is glossy and edges are translucent.

4. Add ½ cup broth, stirring frequently until broth is absorbed before adding next ½ cup. Continue adding broth and stirring until rice is tender and mixture is creamy, about 20 to 25 minutes. Remove from heat.

5. Stir ½ cup cheese, Italian seasoning and salt into risotto. Gently stir in beets. Sprinkle with lemon juice and additional cheese, if desired. Garnish with lemon wedges. Serve immediately.

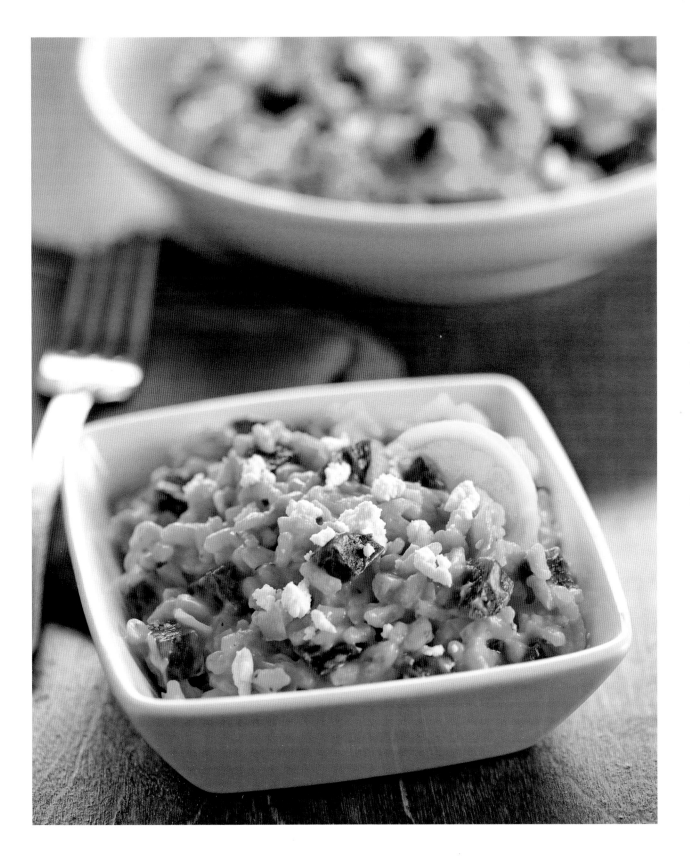

Tuna Steaks with Pineapple Salsa

dairy-free · **nut-free** · **gluten-free**

Makes 4 servings

1 medium tomato, chopped

1 can (8 ounces) pineapple chunks in juice, drained and chopped

2 tablespoons chopped fresh cilantro

1 jalapeño pepper, seeded and minced

1 tablespoon minced red onion

½ teaspoon grated lime peel

2 teaspoons fresh lime juice

4 tuna steaks (4 ounces each)

½ teaspoon salt

⅛ teaspoon black pepper

2 teaspoons extra virgin olive oil

1. For salsa, combine tomato, pineapple, cilantro, jalapeño pepper, onion, lime peel and lime juice in medium bowl.

2. Season tuna with salt and black pepper. Heat oil in large nonstick skillet over medium-high heat. Add tuna; cook 2 to 3 minutes per side for medium-rare or to desired doneness. Serve with salsa.

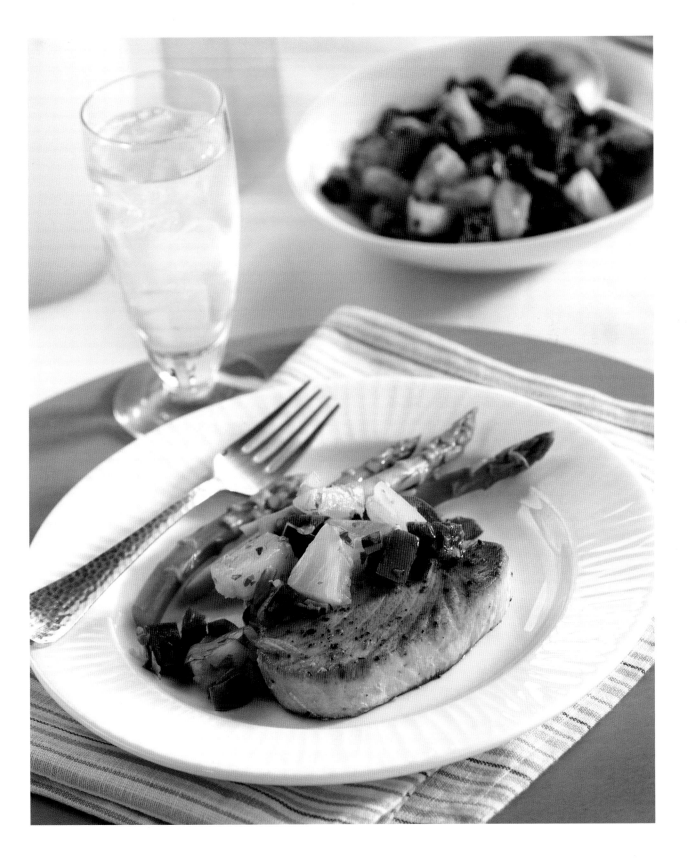

Cold Peanut Noodles with Edamame

vegan · vegetarian · dairy-free · **gluten-free**

Makes 2 servings

½ **(8-ounce) package brown rice pad thai noodles**

3 **tablespoons tamari**

2 **tablespoons dark sesame oil**

2 **tablespoons unseasoned rice vinegar**

1 **tablespoon agave nectar**

1 **tablespoon finely grated fresh ginger**

1 **tablespoon creamy peanut butter**

1 **tablespoon sriracha or hot chile sauce**

2 **teaspoons minced garlic**

½ **cup shelled edamame**

¼ **cup shredded carrots**

¼ **cup sliced green onions**

Chopped peanuts (optional)

1. Prepare noodles according to package directions. Drain and rinse under cold water. Cut noodles into 3-inch lengths. Place in large bowl; set aside.

2. Whisk tamari, oil, vinegar, agave, ginger, peanut butter, sriracha and garlic in small bowl until smooth and well blended. Pour over noodles; toss to coat.

3. Stir in edamame and carrots. Cover and refrigerate at least 30 minutes to allow flavors to develop.

4. Top with green onions and peanuts, if desired, just before serving.

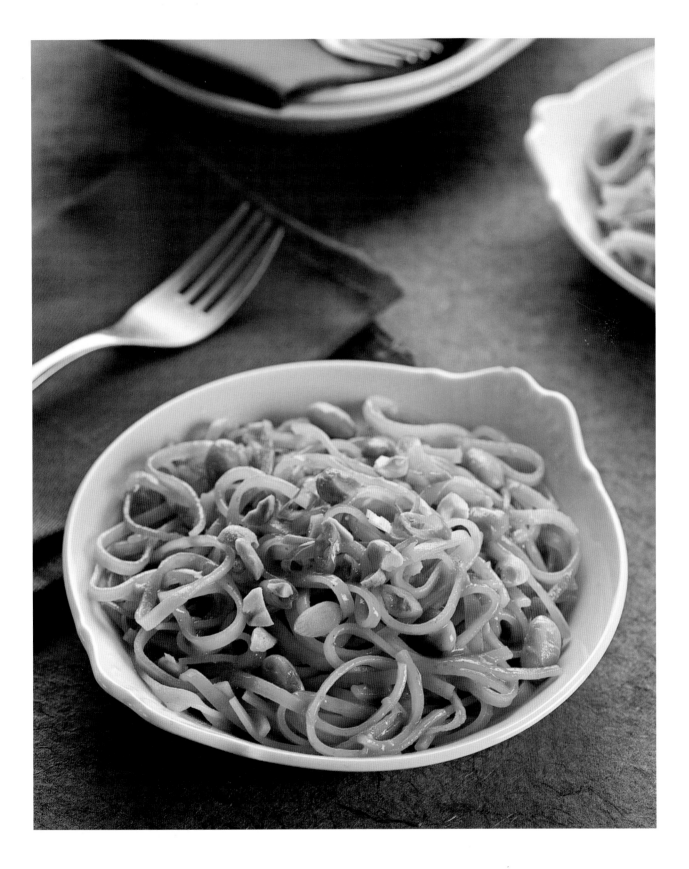

French Carrot Quiche

vegetarian · nut-free

Makes 4 servings

1 pound carrots

1 tablespoon butter

¼ cup chopped green onions

½ teaspoon herbes de Provence

1 cup milk

¼ cup Greek yogurt

½ cup all-purpose flour

2 eggs

½ teaspoon minced fresh thyme

¼ teaspoon ground nutmeg

½ cup shredded Gruyère or Swiss cheese

1. Peel carrots and cut into rounds. Butter four shallow 1-cup baking dishes or one 9-inch quiche dish or shallow casserole. Preheat oven to 350°F.

2. Melt butter in large skillet over medium heat. Add carrots, green onions and herbes de Provence; cook and stir 3 to 4 minutes or until carrots are tender. Spread evenly in prepared dishes.

3. Combine milk and yogurt in medium bowl; gradually whisk in flour. Whisk in eggs, thyme and nutmeg. Pour over carrots; sprinkle with cheese.

4. Bake 20 to 25 minutes for individual quiches (30 to 40 minutes for 9-inch quiche) or until firm. Serve warm or at room temperature.

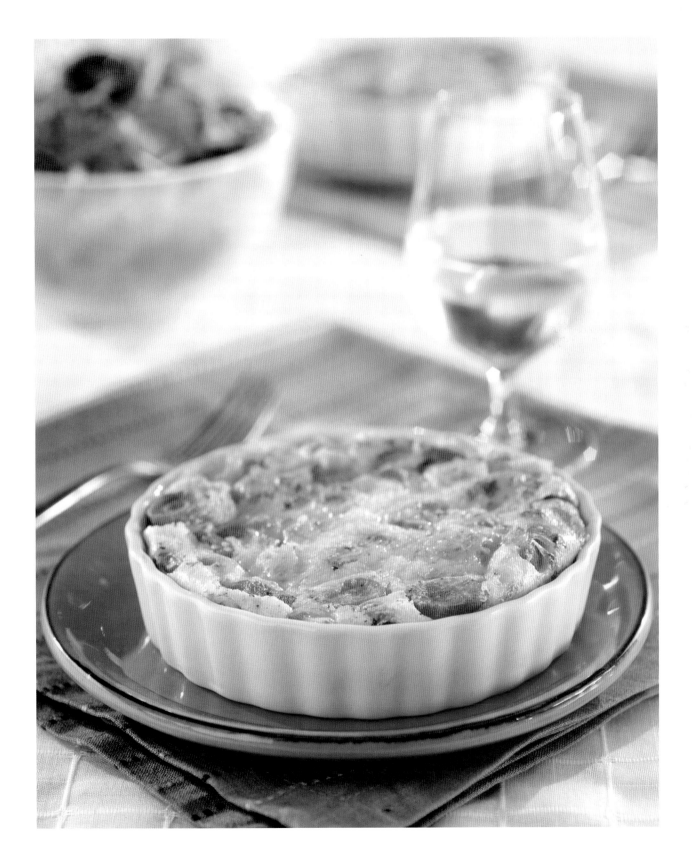

Shanghai Pork Noodle Bowl

dairy-free · **nut-free**

Makes 5 servings

6 ounces uncooked whole wheat spaghetti, broken in half

⅓ cup tamari or soy sauce

2 tablespoons rice vinegar

¼ teaspoon red pepper flakes

2 teaspoons canola oil

1 pound lean pork tenderloin, halved lengthwise and cut into ¼-inch slices

4 cups sliced bok choy

1 can (11 ounces) mandarin orange sections, drained

½ cup sliced green onions

1. Cook noodles according to package directions. Drain and keep warm in large bowl. Stir tamari, vinegar and red pepper flakes in small bowl until blended. Set aside.

2. Heat 1 teaspoon canola oil in large nonstick skillet over medium-high heat. Add half of pork; stir-fry 2 to 3 minutes or until barely pink. Transfer to bowl. Repeat with remaining oil and pork.

3. Add bok choy to skillet; stir-fry 1 to 2 minutes or until wilted. Return pork to skillet. Stir in tamari mixture; cook until heated through.

4. Add pork mixture, orange sections and green onions to pasta; toss until coated.

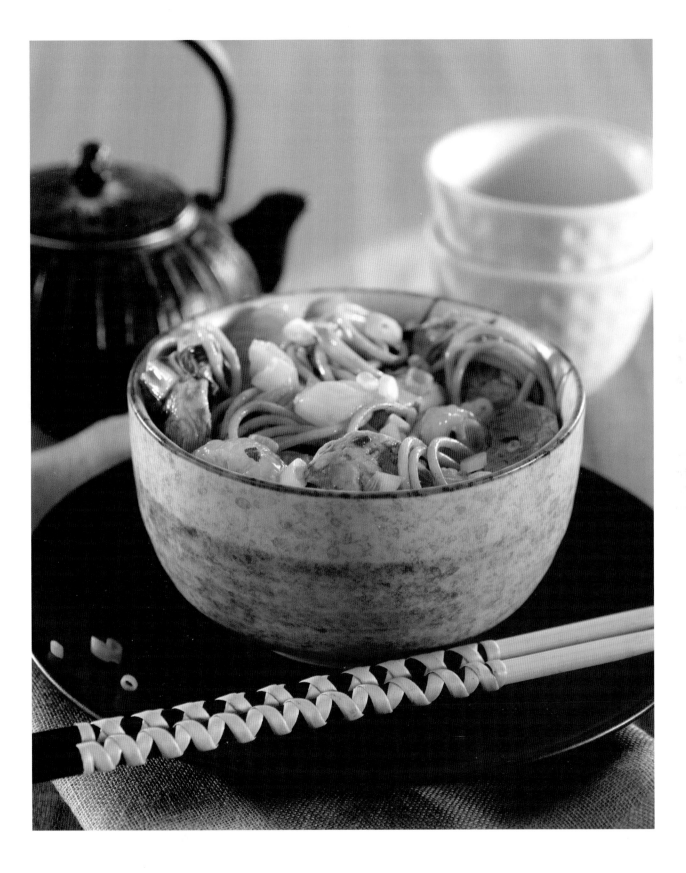

Sweet Potato Gnocchi

vegan · vegetarian · dairy-free · **nut-free** · **gluten-free**

Makes 4 servings

1½ **pounds sweet potatoes (2 or 3 medium)**

¼ **cup sweet rice flour,* plus additional for rolling**

1 **tablespoon fresh lemon juice**

1 **teaspoon salt**

½ **teaspoon xanthan gum**

½ **teaspoon ground nutmeg**

½ **teaspoon black pepper**

2 **to 4 tablespoons extra virgin olive oil**

1 **pound spinach, stemmed**

*Sweet rice flour is usually labeled mochiko (the Japanese term). It is available in the Asian section of large supermarkets, at Asian grocers and online.

1. Preheat oven to 350°F. Bake sweet potatoes 1 hour or until tender. Or pierce sweet potatoes several times with fork and place on microwavable plate. Microwave on HIGH 16 to 18 minutes, rotating halfway through cooking time. Let stand 5 minutes.

2. Cut hot sweet potatoes lengthwise into halves. Scrape pulp from skins into medium bowl. Add ¼ cup rice flour, lemon juice, salt, xanthan gum, nutmeg and pepper; mix well.

3. Heavily dust cutting board or work surface with additional rice flour. Working in batches, scoop portions of dough onto board and roll into ½-inch-thick rope using rice-floured hands. Cut each rope into ¾-inch pieces. Press against tines of fork to make ridges. Place gnocchi on baking sheet; freeze at least 30 minutes.*

4. Heat 1 tablespoon oil in large nonstick skillet. Add gnocchi in single layer and cook until lightly browned and heated through, turning once and adding additional oil as needed to prevent sticking. Keep warm.

5. Add 1 tablespoon oil to skillet. Add spinach; cook and stir 30 seconds or until barely wilted. Serve with gnocchi.

*Gnocchi may be made ahead to this point and frozen for up to 24 hours. For longer storage, transfer frozen gnocchi to covered freezer container.

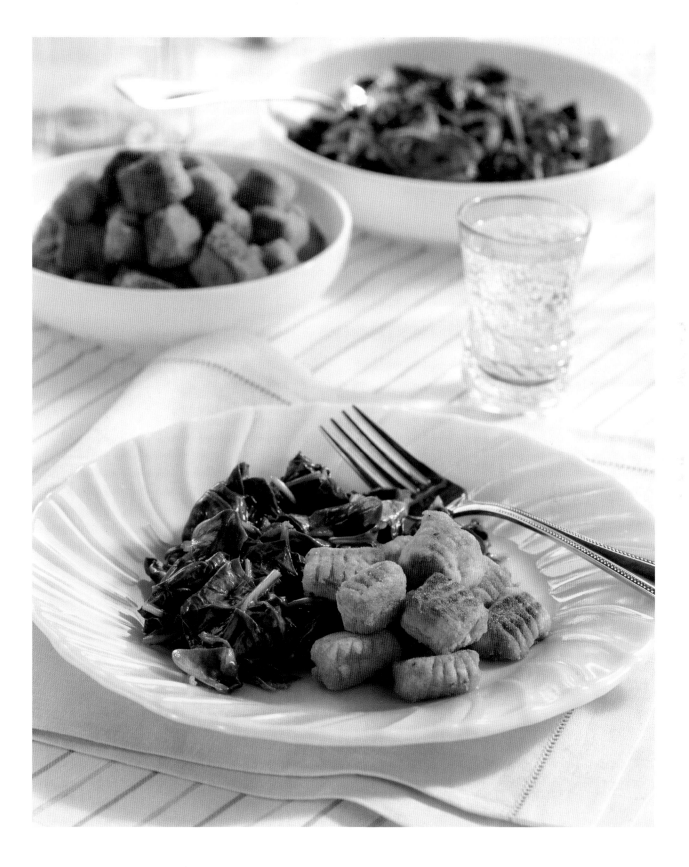

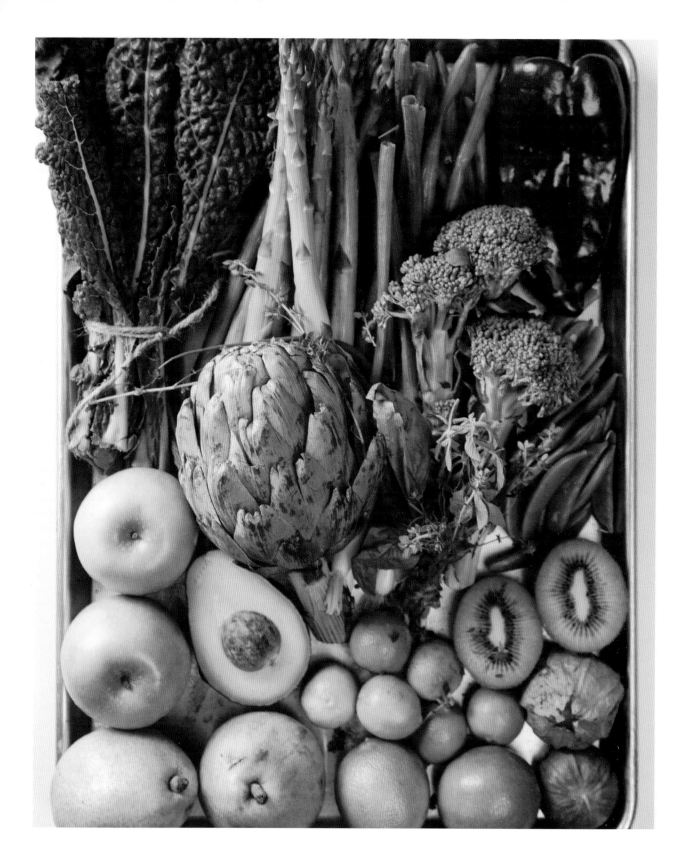

Vegetables & Sides

Glazed Parsnips and Carrots

vegetarian · nut-free · gluten-free

Makes 6 servings

1 **pound parsnips (2 large or 3 medium), quartered lengthwise and cut into sticks**

8 **ounces carrots, quartered lengthwise and cut into sticks**

1 **tablespoon canola oil**

Salt and black pepper

¼ **cup fresh orange juice**

1 **tablespoon butter**

1 **tablespoon honey**

⅛ **teaspoon ground ginger**

1. Preheat oven to 425°F.

2. Spread vegetables in shallow roasting pan. Drizzle with oil and season with salt and pepper; toss to coat. Bake 30 to 35 minutes or until fork-tender.

3. Combine orange juice, butter, honey and ginger in large skillet. Add vegetables; cook and stir over high heat 1 to 2 minutes or until glazed.

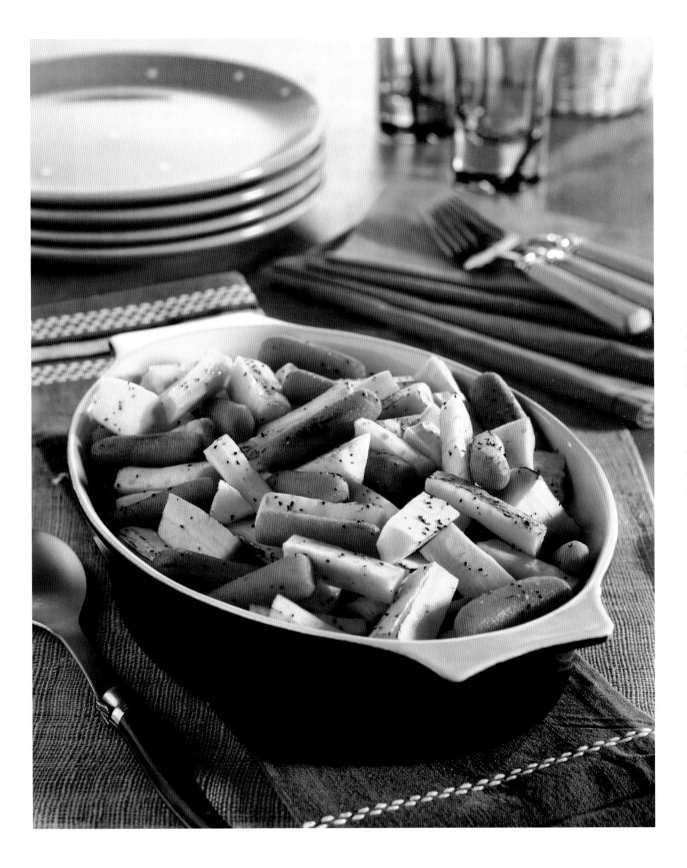

Orange- and Maple-Glazed Beets

vegan · vegetarian · dairy-free · nut-free · gluten-free

Makes 4 servings

4 **medium beets, scrubbed**

2 **teaspoons extra virgin olive oil**

¼ **cup fresh orange juice**

3 **tablespoons balsamic or cider vinegar**

2 **tablespoons maple syrup**

2 **teaspoons grated orange peel, divided**

1 **teaspoon Dijon mustard**

1 **to 2 tablespoons chopped fresh mint (optional)**

Salt and black pepper

1. Preheat oven to 425°F.

2. Place beets in glass baking dish. Drizzle with oil; toss to coat evenly. Cover and bake 45 minutes to 1 hour or until knife inserted into largest beet goes in easily. Let stand until cool enough to handle.

3. Peel and cut beets in half lengthwise; cut into wedges. Return to baking dish.

4. Whisk orange juice, vinegar, maple syrup, 1 teaspoon orange peel and mustard in small bowl until well blended. Pour over beets.

5. Bake 10 to 15 minutes or until heated through and all liquid is absorbed. Sprinkle with remaining 1 teaspoon orange peel and mint, if desired. Season with salt and pepper.

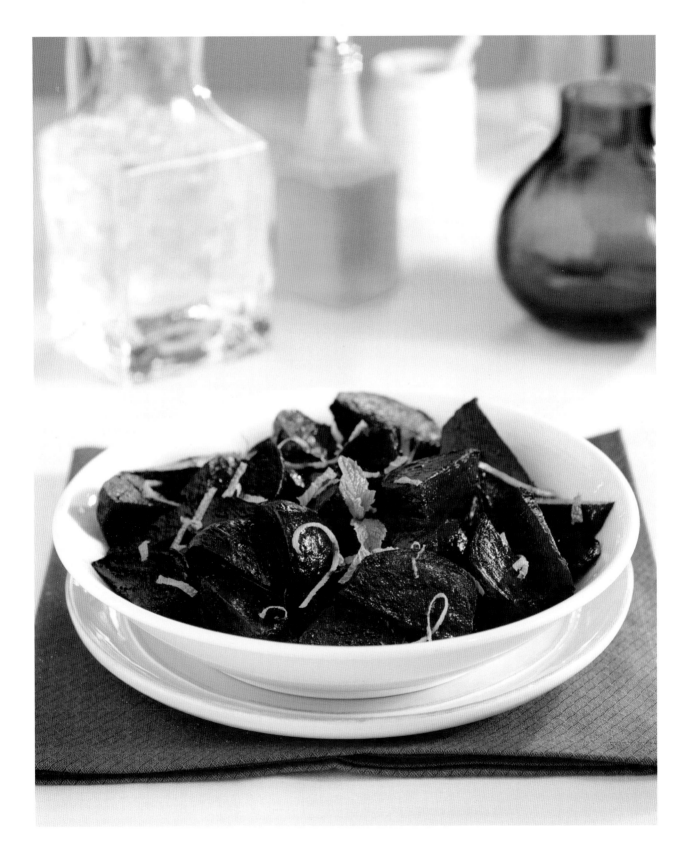

Wheat Berry Apple Salad

vegan · vegetarian · dairy-free

Makes about 6 cups

1 cup uncooked wheat berries (whole wheat kernels)

½ teaspoon salt

1 Granny Smith apple

1 tart red apple

½ cup dried cranberries

⅓ cup chopped walnuts

1 stalk celery, chopped

Grated peel and juice of 1 medium orange

2 tablespoons rice wine vinegar

1½ tablespoons chopped fresh mint

Lettuce leaves (optional)

1. Place wheat berries and salt in large saucepan; cover with 1 inch of water.* Bring to a boil. Stir and reduce heat to low. Cover and cook 45 minutes to 1 hour or until wheat berries are tender but chewy, stirring occasionally. (Add additional water if wheat berries become dry during cooking.) Drain and let cool. (Refrigerate up to 4 days if not using immediately.)

2. Cut apples into bite-size pieces. Combine wheat berries, apples, cranberries, walnuts, celery, orange peel, orange juice, vinegar and mint in large bowl. Cover and refrigerate at least 1 hour to allow flavors to blend. Serve on lettuce leaves, if desired.

To cut cooking time by 20 to 30 minutes, soak wheat berries in water overnight. Drain and cover with 1 inch fresh water before cooking.

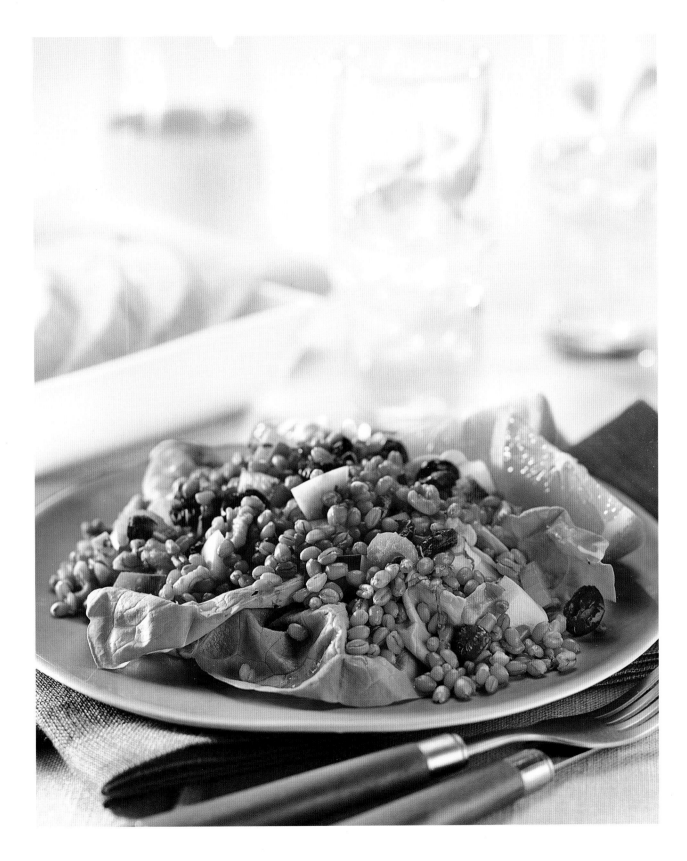

Roasted Asparagus with Orange Glaze

vegan · vegetarian · dairy-free · nut-free · gluten-free

Makes 4 servings

1 pound asparagus, trimmed

2 tablespoons olive oil

2 tablespoons fresh orange juice

½ teaspoon salt

¼ teaspoon black pepper

1½ teaspoons finely shredded or grated orange peel

1. Preheat oven to 425°F.

2. Place asparagus in shallow 1½-quart baking dish. Combine oil and orange juice in small bowl; drizzle over asparagus. Sprinkle with salt and pepper; roll to coat.

3. Roast 12 minutes for medium-sized asparagus or until asparagus is crisp-tender. Garnish with orange peel.

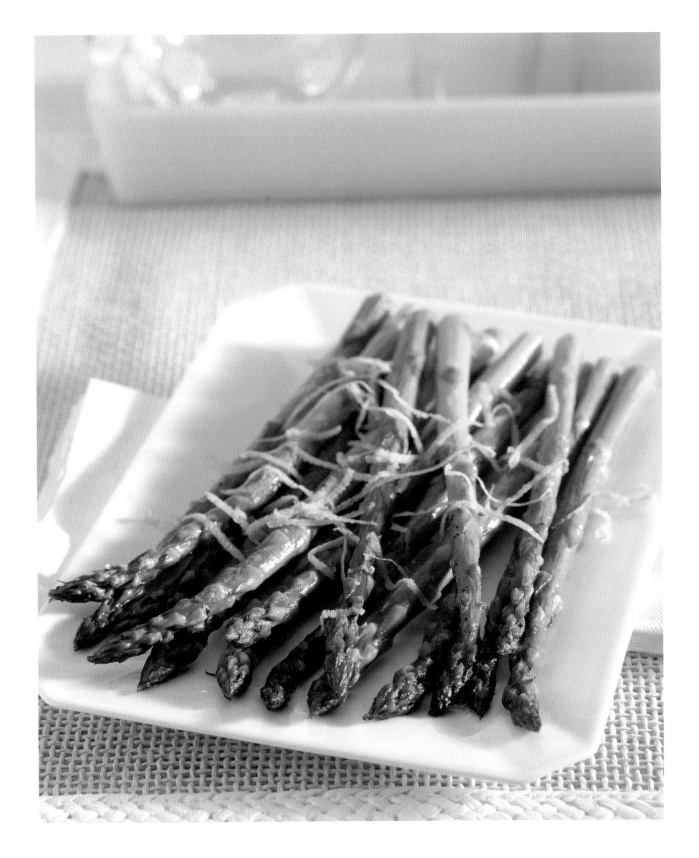

Roasted Cremini Mushrooms

vegan · vegetarian · dairy-free **· nut-free · gluten-free**

Makes 4 servings

1 **pound cremini mushrooms, stems trimmed, halved**

½ **cup sliced shallots**

1 **tablespoon extra virgin olive oil**

½ **teaspoon coarse salt**

½ **teaspoon dried rosemary**

¼ **teaspoon black pepper**

1. Preheat oven to 400°F.

2. Spread mushrooms and shallots on rimmed baking sheet. Whisk oil, salt, rosemary and pepper in small bowl. Pour over mushrooms and shallots; toss to coat evenly. Arrange in single layer on baking sheet.

3. Bake 15 to 18 minutes or until mushrooms are browned and tender.

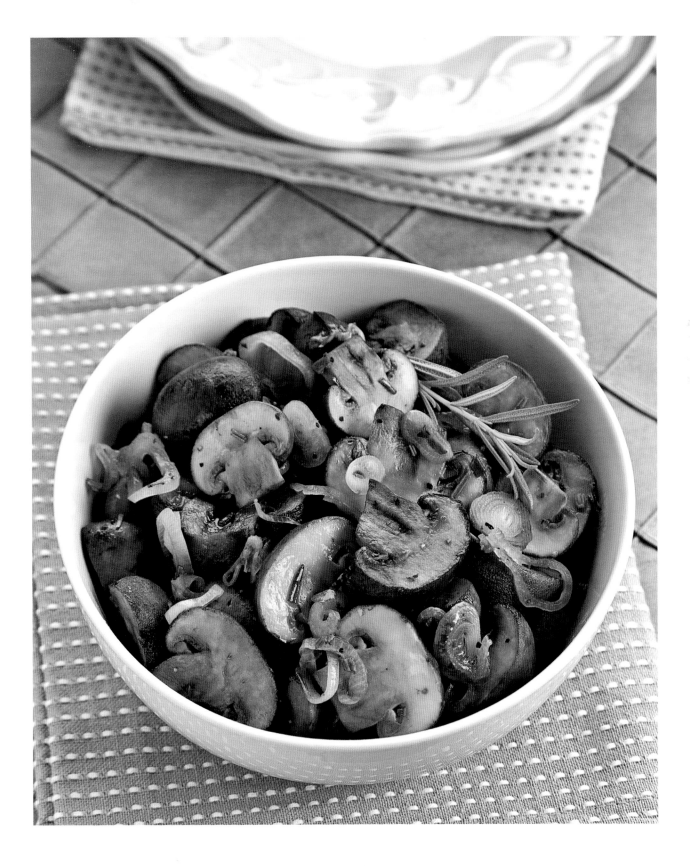

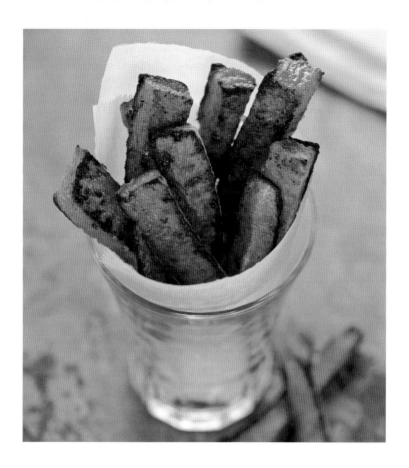

Butternut Squash Oven Fries

vegan · vegetarian · dairy-free · nut-free · gluten-free

Makes 4 servings

½ **teaspoon garlic powder**

¼ **teaspoon salt**

¼ **teaspoon ground red pepper**

1 **butternut squash (about 2½ pounds), peeled, seeded and cut into thin 2-inch-long sticks**

2 **teaspoons canola oil**

1. Preheat oven to 425°F. Combine garlic powder, salt and red pepper in small bowl.

2. Place squash on baking sheet. Drizzle with oil and sprinkle with seasoning mix; gently toss to coat. Arrange in single layer.

3. Bake 20 to 25 minutes or until squash just begins to brown, stirring frequently.

4. Preheat broiler. Broil 3 to 5 minutes or until fries are browned and crisp. Spread on paper towels to cool slightly before serving.

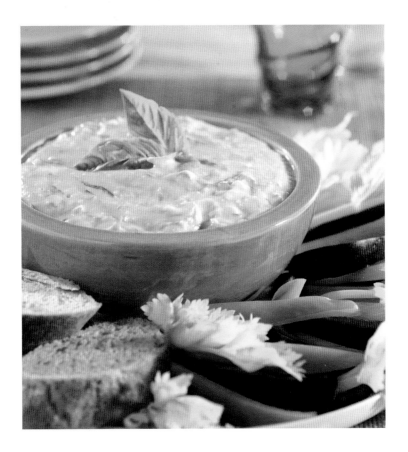

Basil Cannellini Dip

vegan · **vegetarian** · *dairy-free* · **nut-free**

Makes about 1½ cups

1 **can (about 15 ounces) cannellini or Great Northern beans**

1 **clove garlic**

2 **tablespoons extra virgin olive oil**

3 **tablespoons chopped fresh basil**

Salt and black pepper

Bell pepper sticks and whole g rain French bread

1. Drain beans, reserving ¼ cup liquid. Rinse beans and drain well.

2. With motor running, drop garlic clove through feed tube of food processor; process until finely chopped. Stop processor; add beans, reserved liquid and oil. Process until smooth.

3. Stir in basil. Season with salt and pepper.

Note: To make this dish gluten-free, skip the bread and serve with rice crackers or additional cut-up vegetables.

Spicy Roasted Chickpeas

vegan · vegetarian · dairy-free · nut-free · gluten-free

Makes 2 cups

1 **can (about 15 ounces) chickpeas, rinsed and drained**

3 **tablespoons extra virgin olive oil**

½ **teaspoon salt**

½ **teaspoon black pepper**

1 **tablespoon chili powder**

⅛ **to ¼ teaspoon ground red pepper**

1 **lime, cut into wedges**

1. Preheat oven to 400°F.

2. Combine chickpeas, oil, salt and black pepper in large bowl. Spread in single layer on 15×10-inch jelly-roll pan.

3. Bake 15 minutes or until chickpeas begin to brown, shaking pan twice. Sprinkle with chili powder and red pepper. Bake 5 minutes or until dark golden-red. Cool slightly; serve with lime wedges.

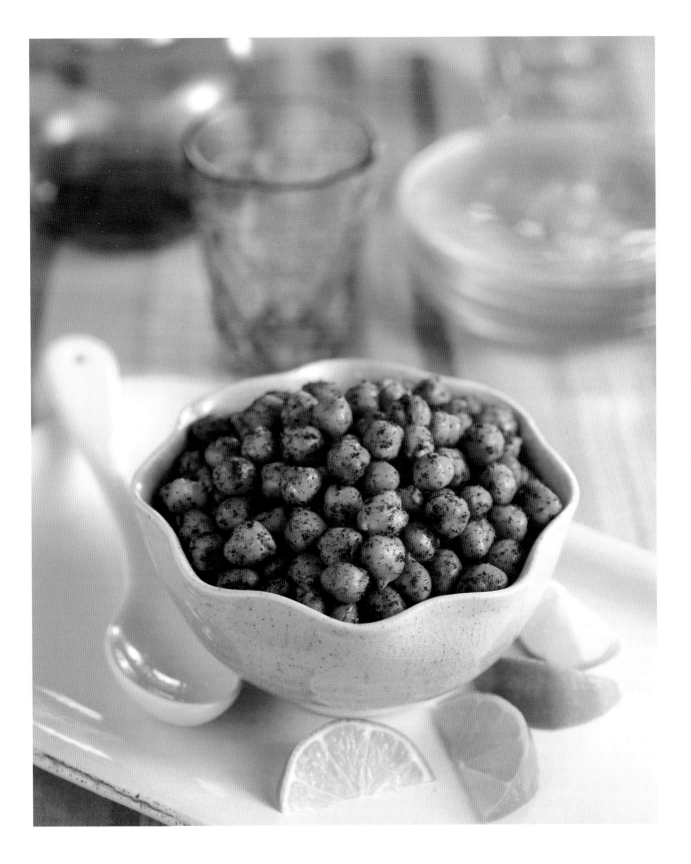

Beans and Greens with Curry

vegan · vegetarian · *dairy-free* · nut-free · gluten-free

Makes 8 servings

1 cup adzuki beans*

4 cups plus 2 tablespoons cold water, plus additional for soaking

2 pounds Swiss chard or kale

1 tablespoon extra virgin olive oil

½ cup diced white onion

2 cloves garlic, minced

2 teaspoons sweet or spicy curry powder

¼ teaspoon salt

¼ teaspoon freshly ground black pepper

Adzuki beans are small reddish beans with a sweet flavor and high protein content. They are used in Japanese cooking and can be found at natural food markets.

1. Soak beans overnight in enough water to cover by at least 2 inches. Drain beans and rinse well.

2. Place beans in large saucepan with 4 cups water; bring to a boil. Reduce heat and simmer 1 hour or until beans are tender. Drain beans; set aside.

3. Remove stems and ribs from chard and tear into large pieces.

4. Heat oil in large deep skillet over medium heat. Add onion and garlic; cook and stir 5 minutes or until onion is soft and translucent. Add curry powder; cook and stir 30 seconds or until slightly toasted and aromatic.

5. Add greens to skillet; sprinkle with 2 tablespoons water. Cook 5 minutes or until wilted.

6. Add beans to chard mixture; cook and stir until heated through. Season with salt and pepper.

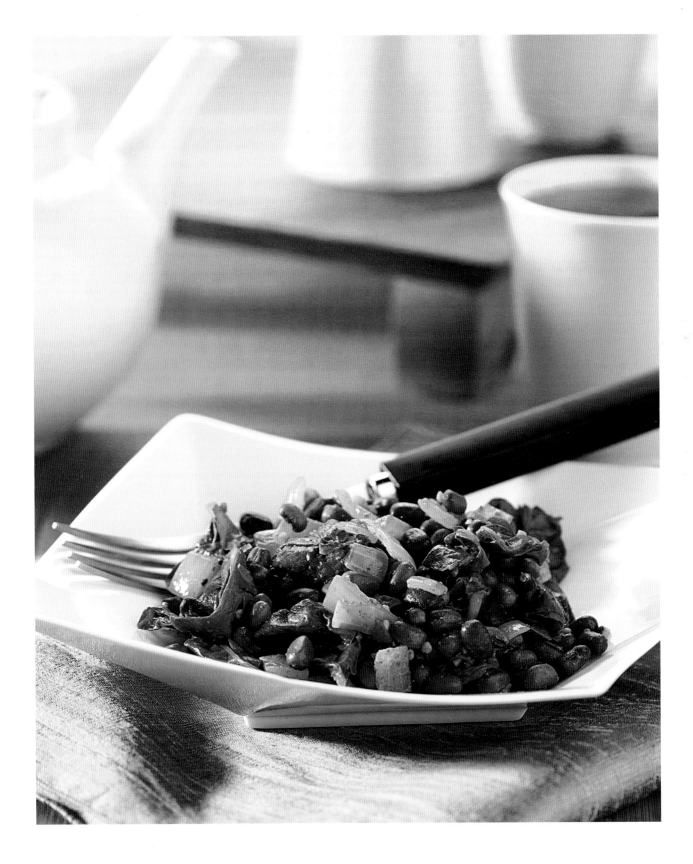

White Bean and Spinach Bruschetta

vegan · vegetarian · dairy-free · nut-free

Makes 16 servings

1 can (about 15 ounces) Great Northern or cannellini beans, rinsed and drained

4 tablespoons extra virgin olive oil, divided

2 cloves garlic, minced

½ teaspoon salt, divided

½ teaspoon black pepper, divided

6 cups loosely packed spinach, finely chopped

1 tablespoon red wine vinegar

16 slices whole grain baguette

1. Purée beans in food processor, adding 1 to 2 tablespoons water for smoother texture, if desired. Transfer to medium bowl.

2. Heat 1 tablespoon oil in medium skillet. Add garlic; cook and stir 1 minute. Remove from heat; add ¼ teaspoon salt and ¼ teaspoon pepper. Stir into beans.

3. Heat 1 tablespoon oil in same skillet over medium heat. Add spinach; cook 2 to 3 minutes or until wilted. Stir in vinegar, remaining ¼ teaspoon salt and ¼ teaspoon pepper. Remove from heat.

4. Preheat broiler. Brush baguette slices with remaining 2 tablespoons oil. Broil until bread is golden brown and crisp. Top with bean purée and spinach. Serve immediately.

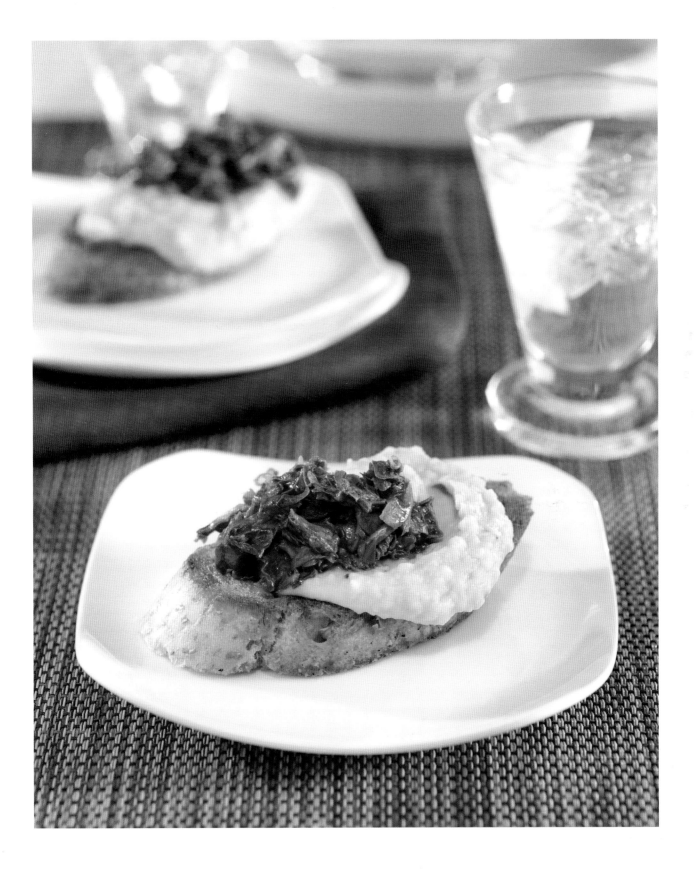

Zucchini Ribbon Salad

vegetarian · **gluten-free**

Makes 2 servings

2 **medium zucchini**

2 **tablespoons chopped sun-dried tomatoes (not packed in oil)**

2 **teaspoons extra virgin olive oil**

1 **teaspoon fresh lemon juice**

1 **teaspoon white wine vinegar**

⅛ **teaspoon salt**

2 **tablespoons shredded Parmesan cheese**

1 **tablespoon pine nuts, toasted***

*To toast pine nuts, spread in single layer in heavy skillet. Cook over medium heat 1 to 2 minutes or until nuts are lightly browned, stirring frequently.

1. Peel zucchini lengthwise into ribbons using vegetable peeler until seeds are visible. Combine zucchini ribbons and sun-dried tomatoes in medium bowl.

2. Whisk oil, lemon juice, vinegar and salt in small bowl until well blended. Drizzle over zucchini and tomatoes; gently toss to coat.

3. Divide salad evenly between two serving bowls. Top with cheese and pine nuts. Serve immediately.

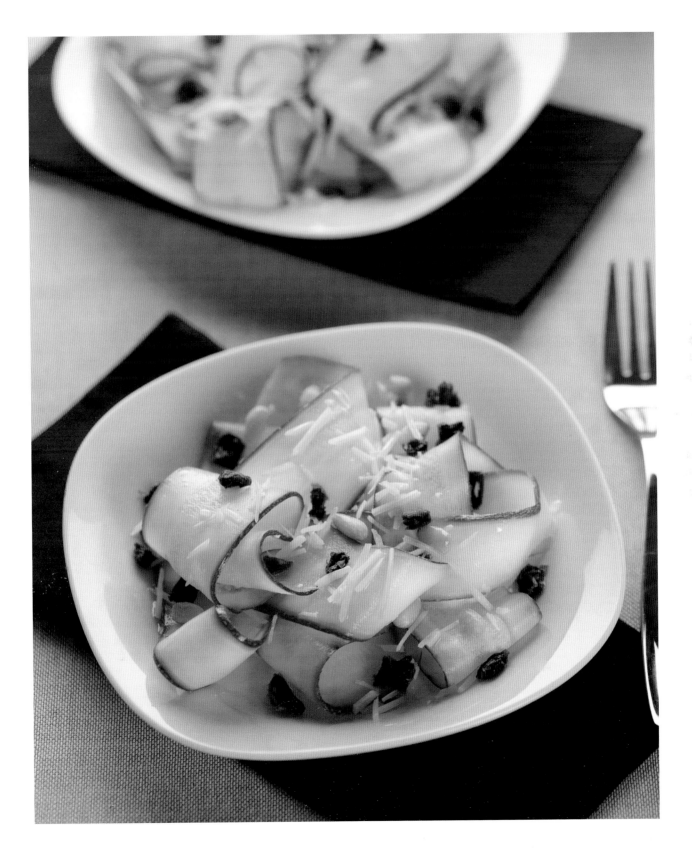

Warm Moroccan-Style Bean Dip

vegetarian • nut-free

Makes 4 to 6 servings

2 teaspoons canola oil

1 onion, chopped

2 cloves garlic, minced

2 cans (about 15 ounces each) cannellini beans, rinsed and drained

¾ cup canned diced tomatoes, drained

½ teaspoon ground turmeric (optional)

¼ teaspoon salt

¼ teaspoon ground cumin

¼ teaspoon ground cinnamon

¼ teaspoon paprika

¼ teaspoon black pepper

⅛ teaspoon ground cloves

⅛ teaspoon ground red pepper

2 tablespoons plain yogurt

1 tablespoon water

¼ teaspoon dried mint (optional)

Warm whole wheat pita bread rounds, cut into wedges

1. Heat oil in small skillet over medium-high heat. Add onion; cook and stir 5 minutes or until translucent. Add garlic; cook and stir 30 seconds. Transfer to slow cooker. Stir in beans, tomatoes, turmeric, if desired, salt, cumin, cinnamon, paprika, black pepper, cloves and red pepper. Cover; cook on LOW 6 hours.

2. Transfer to food processor or blender; pulse until coarsely chopped. (Or use immersion blender.) Transfer to serving bowl.

3. Whisk yogurt and cold water in small bowl; drizzle over bean dip. Garnish with mint and serve with pita bread wedges.

Note: To make this dish gluten-free, omit the pita bread and serve with bell pepper wedges, carrot sticks or apple wedges.

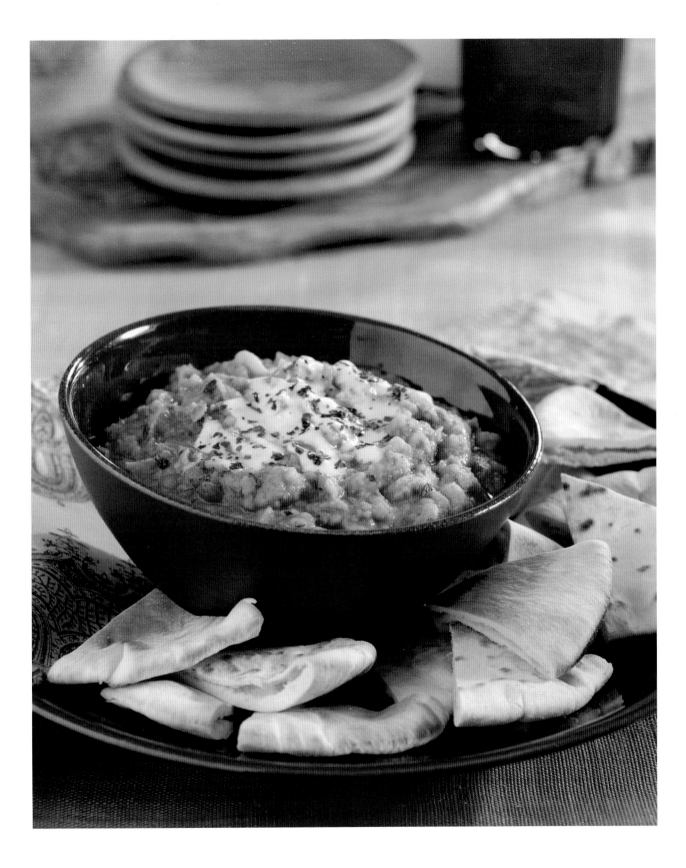

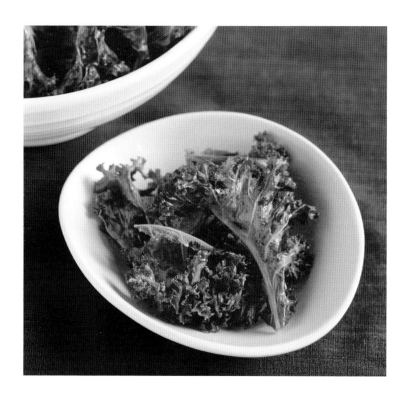

Kale Chips

vegan · **vegetarian** · dairy-free · **nut-free** · **gluten-free**

Makes 6 servings

1 **large bunch kale (about
   1 pound)**

1 **to 2 tablespoons extra
   virgin olive oil**

1 **teaspoon garlic salt or
   other seasoned salt**

1. Preheat oven to 350°F. Line baking sheets with
parchment paper.

2. Wash kale and pat dry with paper towels.
Remove center ribs and stems; discard. Cut leaves
into 2- to 3-inch-wide pieces.

3. Combine kale, oil and garlic salt in large bowl;
toss to coat. Spread on prepared baking sheets.

4. Bake 10 to 15 minutes or until edges are lightly
browned and leaves are crisp.* Cool completely on
baking sheets. Store in airtight container.

*If the leaves are lightly browned but not crisp, turn
oven off and let chips stand in oven until crisp, about 10
minutes. Do not keep the oven on as the chips will burn
easily.*

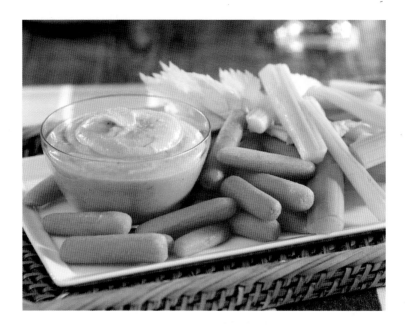

Hot and Spicy Hummus

vegetarian · nut-free · gluten-free

Makes 1¼ cups

1 **can (about 15 ounces) pinto beans, rinsed and drained**

1 **clove garlic**

1 **teaspoon canned chipotle peppers in adobo sauce**

¼ **cup plain yogurt**

2 **teaspoons fresh lemon juice**

1 **teaspoon extra virgin olive oil**

½ **teaspoon ground cumin**

⅜ **teaspoon salt**

¼ **teaspoon black pepper**

2 **to 3 tablespoons water (optional)**

Celery sticks, carrot sticks and/or blanched broccoli and cauliflower florets

1. Combine beans, chipotle pepper, chile, yogurt, lemon juice, oil, cumin, salt and black pepper in food processor or blender. Process until puréed, scraping down side of bowl occasionally. Add 2 to 3 tablespoons water, if necessary, to reach desired consistency.

2. Transfer to serving bowl. Serve with vegetables.

Potato-Zucchini Pancakes with Warm Corn Salsa

vegetarian · dairy-free · **nut-free** · **gluten-free**

Makes 6 servings

Warm Corn Salsa (recipe follows)

2 **cups shredded russet potatoes, squeezed dry**

1½ **cups shredded zucchini, squeezed dry**

2 **eggs, lightly beaten**

¼ **cup all-purpose flour**

2 **tablespoons chopped onion**

2 **tablespoons chopped green bell pepper**

¼ **teaspoon salt**

⅛ **teaspoon black pepper**

2 **tablespoons canola oil**

1. Prepare Warm Corn Salsa; keep warm.

2. Combine potatoes, zucchini, eggs, flour, onion, bell pepper, salt and black pepper in medium bowl; gently mix.

3. Heat 1 tablespoon oil in large skillet over medium-high heat. Working in batches, drop ¼ cupfuls of potato mixture into skillet. Cook 3 minutes per side or until golden brown, adding additional oil if needed. Serve with salsa.

Warm Corn Salsa

vegan · vegetarian · dairy-free · **nut-free** · **gluten-free**

Makes 3 cups

---

1 **tablespoon extra virgin olive oil**

2 **tablespoons chopped onion**

2 **tablespoons finely chopped green bell pepper**

2 **cups corn**

1 **cup chunky salsa**

2 **teaspoons chopped fresh cilantro**

1. Heat oil in medium skillet. Add onion and bell pepper; cook and stir 3 minutes or until crisp-tender.

2. Add corn, salsa and cilantro. Reduce heat to medium-low; cook 5 minutes or until heated through.

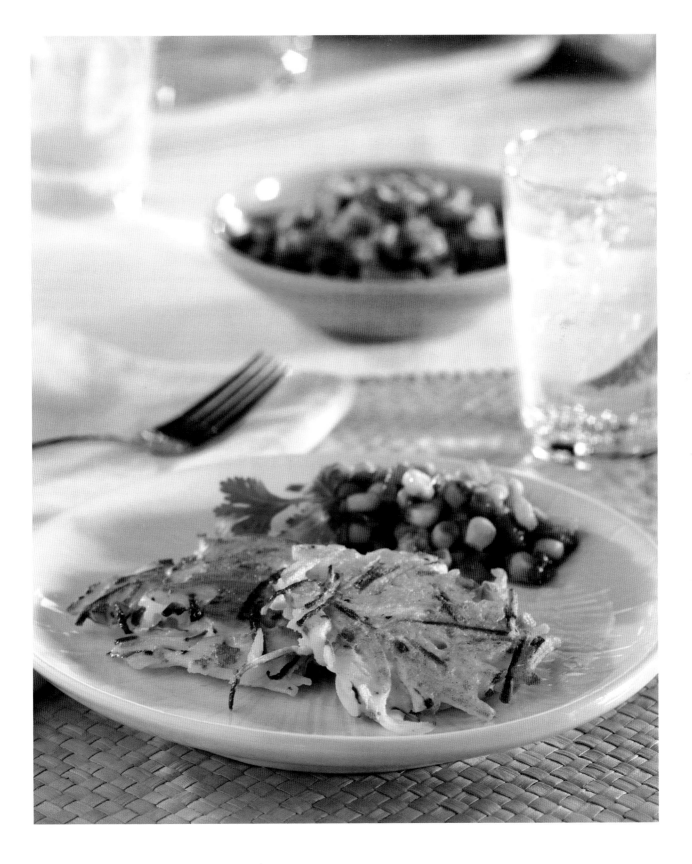

Zucchini with Toasted Chickpea Flour

vegan • **vegetarian** • *dairy-free* • **nut-free** • **gluten-free**

Makes 4 servings

½ **cup sifted chickpea flour**

3 **tablespoons extra virgin olive oil**

3 **teaspoons minced garlic**

2 **medium zucchini, cut into ½-inch-thick circles or half circles**

2 **medium summer squash, cut into ½-inch-thick circles or half circles**

1 **teaspoon salt**

½ **teaspoon black pepper**

½ **cup water**

1. Heat small skillet over medium-high heat; add chickpea flour. Cook and stir 3 to 4 minutes until fragrant and slightly darker in color. Remove from skillet; set aside.

2. Heat oil in large skillet over medium-high heat. Add garlic; cook and stir 1 minute or until fragrant. Add zucchini, squash, salt and pepper; cook and stir 5 minutes or until beginning to soften.

3. Stir chickpea flour into skillet to coat vegetables. Pour in water; cook and stir 2 to 3 minutes or until moist crumbs form, scraping bottom of skillet frequently to prevent sticking and scrape up brown bits.

Note: Using chickpea flour to add substance and nutrition to vegetable dishes is a method adapted from Indian cuisine. The flour forms delicious, nutty crumbs that stick to the vegetables. The same method can be used with other vegetables as well.

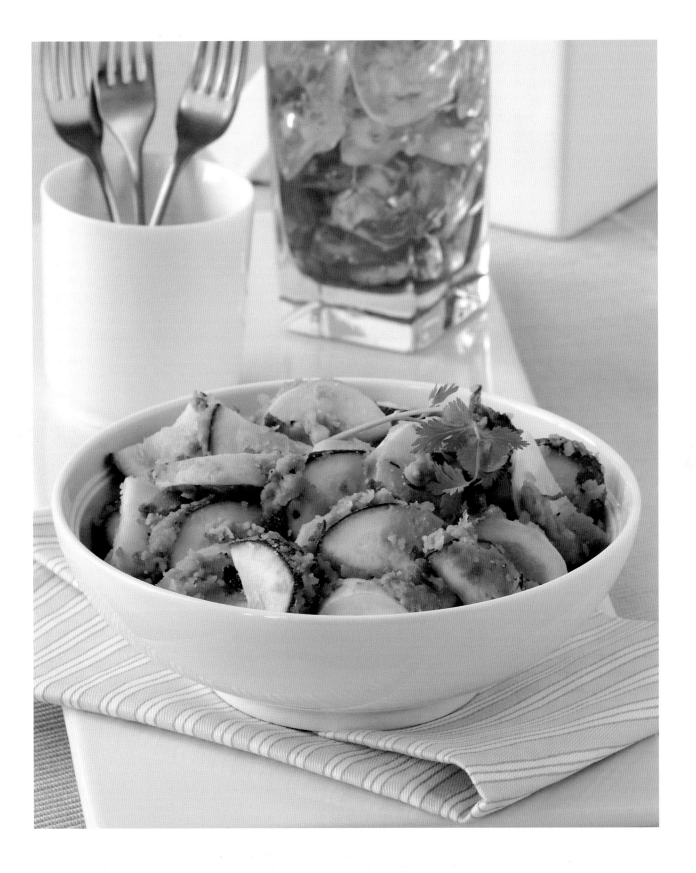

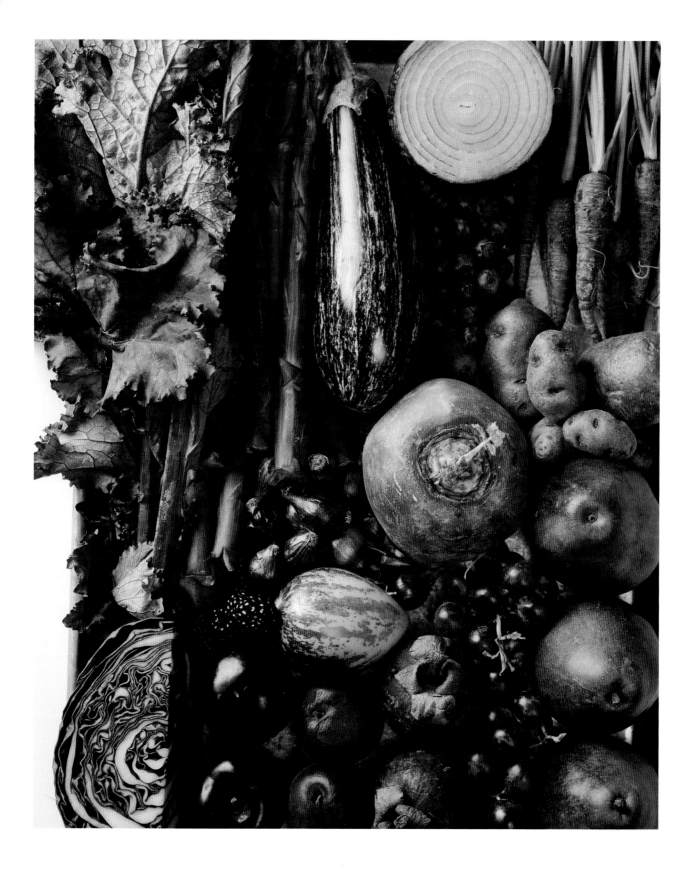

Fruit Finales

Peanut Butter Berry Bars

vegan · vegetarian · dairy-free · **gluten-free**

Makes 16 servings

2 cups quick oats

½ cup natural peanut butter

½ cup bittersweet chocolate chips or finely chopped bittersweet chocolate, divided

¼ cup packed brown sugar

¼ cup canola oil, divided

1 teaspoon ground cinnamon

¾ cup finely chopped fresh strawberries

Sliced strawberries (optional)

1. Heat large skillet over medium-high heat. Add oats; cook and stir 6 minutes or until lightly browned and fragrant. Remove from skillet; set aside.

2. Combine peanut butter, 5 tablespoons chocolate chips, brown sugar, 2½ tablespoons oil and cinnamon in same skillet. Cook and stir over low heat until melted and smooth. Remove from heat. Add oats; stir until well blended. Press mixture evenly into 9-inch square baking pan using rubber spatula. Freeze 15 minutes to cool. Sprinkle with chopped strawberries.

3. Place remaining chocolate chips and oil in small saucepan; cook over low heat until chips are melted, stirring constantly. Drizzle over strawberries. Cover with foil and freeze at least 2 hours.

4. Let stand 10 minutes at room temperature. Cut into squares and garnish with sliced strawberries. Freeze leftovers.

Note: To make sure this recipe is gluten-free and vegan, buy gluten-free oats (oats that are not processed in a facility that also processes gluten products). Also, look for chocolate that does not contain any milk products.

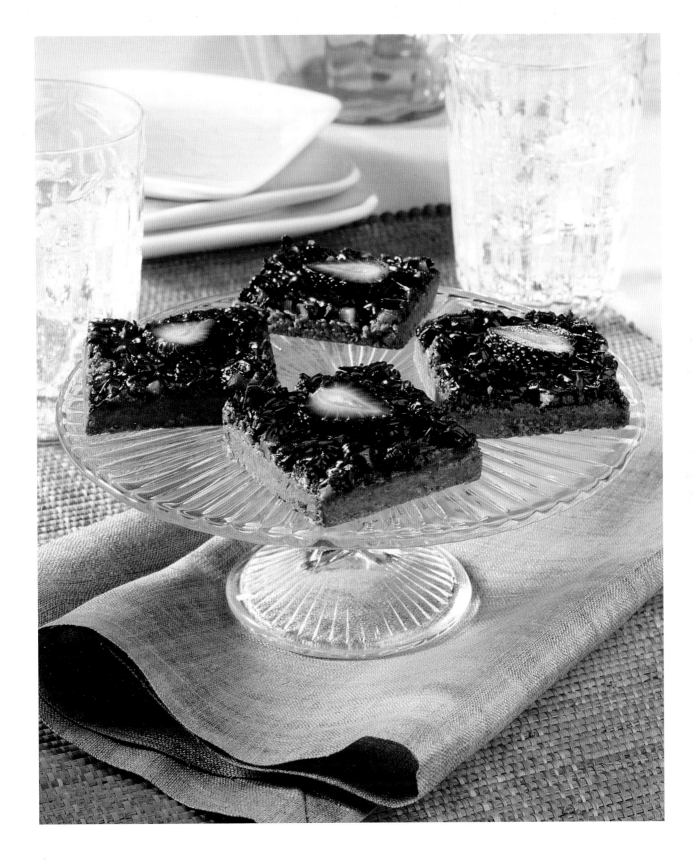

Fruit Salad
with Creamy Banana Dressing

vegetarian · nut-free · gluten-free

Makes 8 servings

2 cups fresh pineapple
    chunks

1 cup cantaloupe cubes

1 cup honeydew melon cubes

1 cup fresh blackberries

1 cup sliced fresh
    strawberries

1 cup seedless red grapes

1 medium apple, diced

2 medium ripe bananas

½ cup Greek yogurt

2 tablespoons honey

1 tablespoon fresh lemon
    juice

¼ teaspoon ground nutmeg

1. Combine pineapple, cantaloupe, honeydew, blackberries, strawberries, grapes and apple in large bowl; gently mix.

2. Combine bananas, yogurt, honey, lemon juice and nutmeg in blender or food processor; blend until smooth.

3. Pour dressing over fruit mixture; stir until evenly coated.

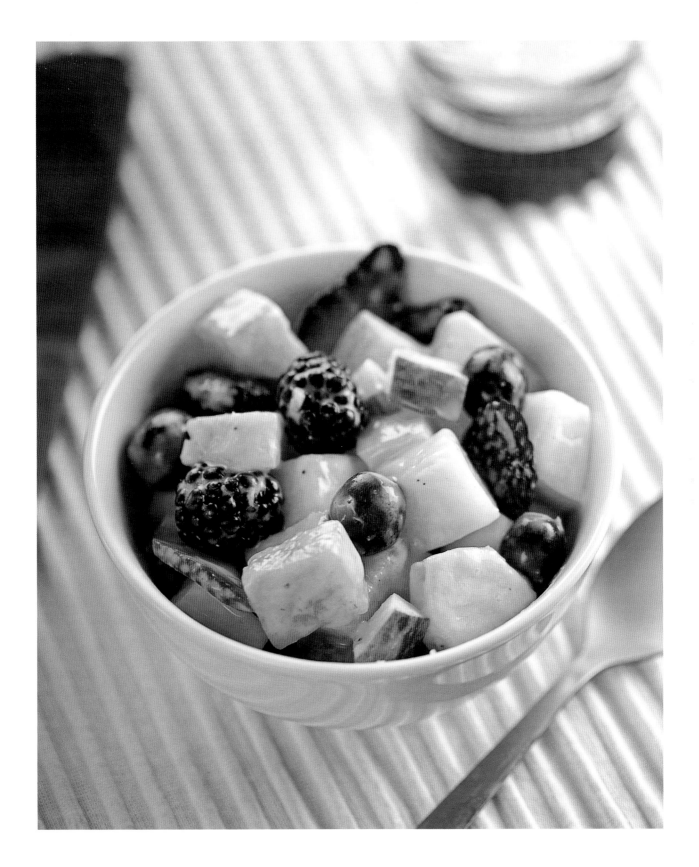

Strawberry-Banana Granité

vegetarian · dairy-free · **nut-free** · **gluten-free**

Makes 5 servings

2 ripe medium bananas, peeled and sliced (about 2 cups)

2 cups frozen strawberries

2 tablespoons honey

1. Place banana slices in resealable freezer food storage bag; freeze until firm.

2. Combine bananas and strawberries in food processor or blender; let stand 10 minutes to soften slightly.

3. Add honey to mixture. Remove plunger from top of food processor to allow air to be incorporated. Process until smooth, scraping down side of bowl frequently. Serve immediately.

Note: Granité can be transferred to airtight container and frozen up to 1 month. Let stand at room temperature 10 minutes to soften slightly before serving.

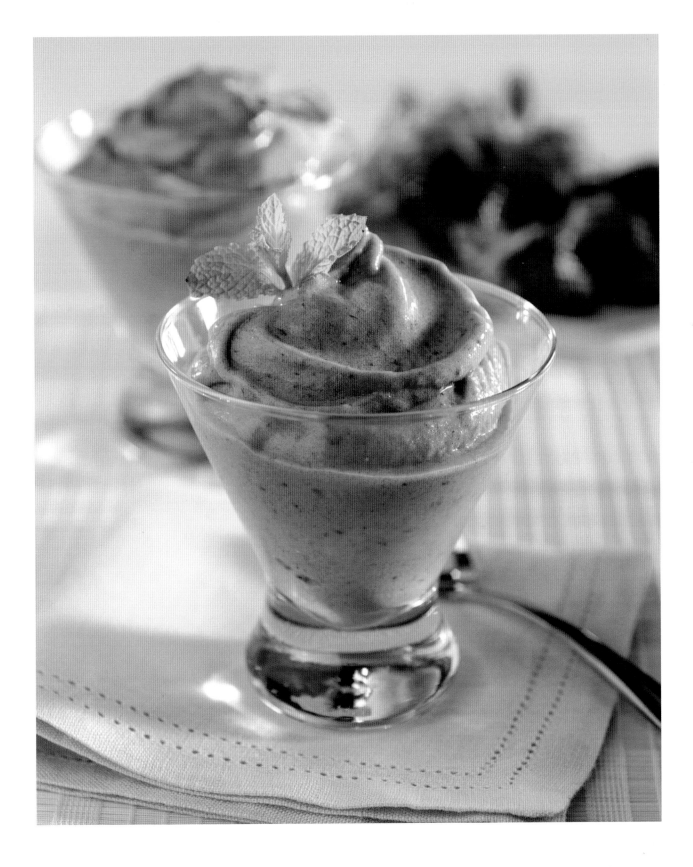

Autumn Fruit Crisp

vegan · vegetarian · dairy-free · nut-free

Makes 6 servings

2 **tart apples, peeled and sliced (1 pound)**

1 **pear, peeled and sliced**

⅓ **cup old-fashioned oats**

¼ **cup packed brown sugar**

2 **tablespoons whole wheat flour**

½ **teaspoon ground cinnamon**

2 **tablespoons coconut oil**

1. Preheat oven to 350°F. Grease 8-inch square baking dish.

2. Combine apples and pear in prepared baking dish. Combine oats, brown sugar, flour and cinnamon in medium bowl; mix well. Cut in coconut oil with pastry blender or two knives until mixture resembles coarse crumbs. Sprinkle evenly over fruit mixture.

3. Bake 35 to 40 minutes or until fruit is tender and topping is lightly browned.

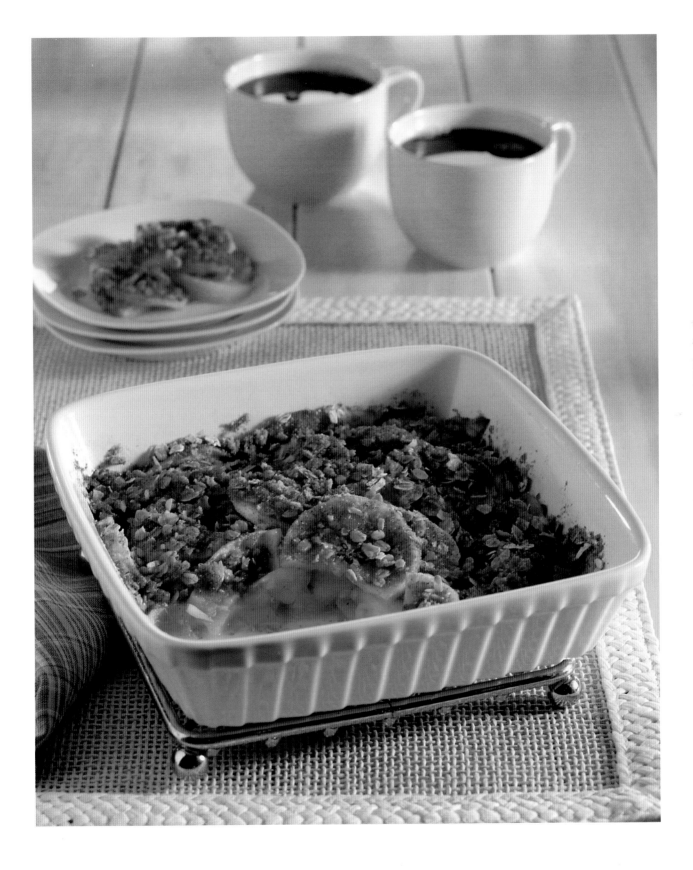

Yogurt Custard with Blueberries

vegetarian · gluten-free

Makes 1 serving

1 **container (6 ounces) plain yogurt**

2 **teaspoons honey**

⅛ **teaspoon ground nutmeg**

½ **cup fresh blueberries**

1 **tablespoon all-fruit blueberry preserves**

1 **tablespoon sliced almonds, toasted**

1. Line fine-mesh sieve with two layers of cheesecloth or paper towels. Add yogurt and place sieve over bowl. Refrigerate 20 minutes to drain and thicken.

2. Combine yogurt, honey and nutmeg in small bowl. Combine blueberries and preserves in small bowl; spoon over yogurt. Top with almonds.

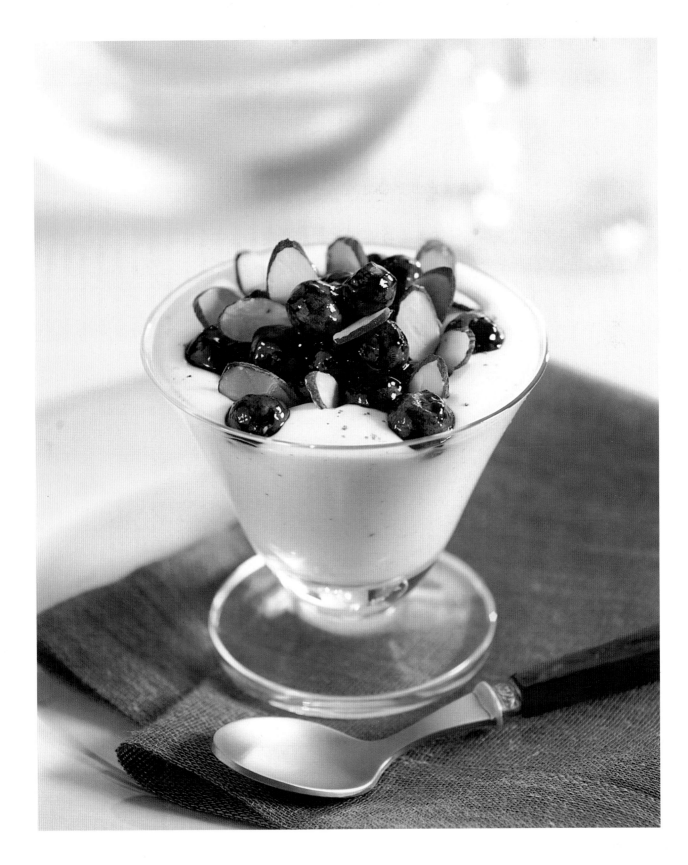

Berry-Quinoa Parfaits

vegetarian · nut-free · gluten-free

Makes 6 servings

⅔ **cup uncooked quinoa**

2 **cups plus 2 tablespoons soymilk, divided**

⅛ **teaspoon salt**

3 **tablespoons honey**

1 **egg**

1½ **teaspoons vanilla**

2 **cups sliced fresh strawberries**

¼ **cup yogurt**

Ground cinnamon (optional)

1. Place quinoa in fine-mesh strainer; rinse well under cold running water. Combine quinoa, 2 cups soymilk and salt in medium saucepan. Bring to a simmer over medium heat. Reduce heat to medium-low; simmer, uncovered, 20 to 25 minutes or until quinoa is tender, stirring frequently.

2. Whisk remaining 2 tablespoons soymilk, honey, egg and vanilla in medium bowl until well blended. Gradually whisk ½ cup hot quinoa mixture into egg mixture, then whisk mixture back into saucepan. Cook over medium heat 3 to 5 minutes or until bubbly and thickened, stirring constantly. Remove from heat; let cool 30 minutes.

3. Layer quinoa mixture and strawberries in six parfait dishes. Top with dollop of yogurt and sprinkle with cinnamon, if desired.

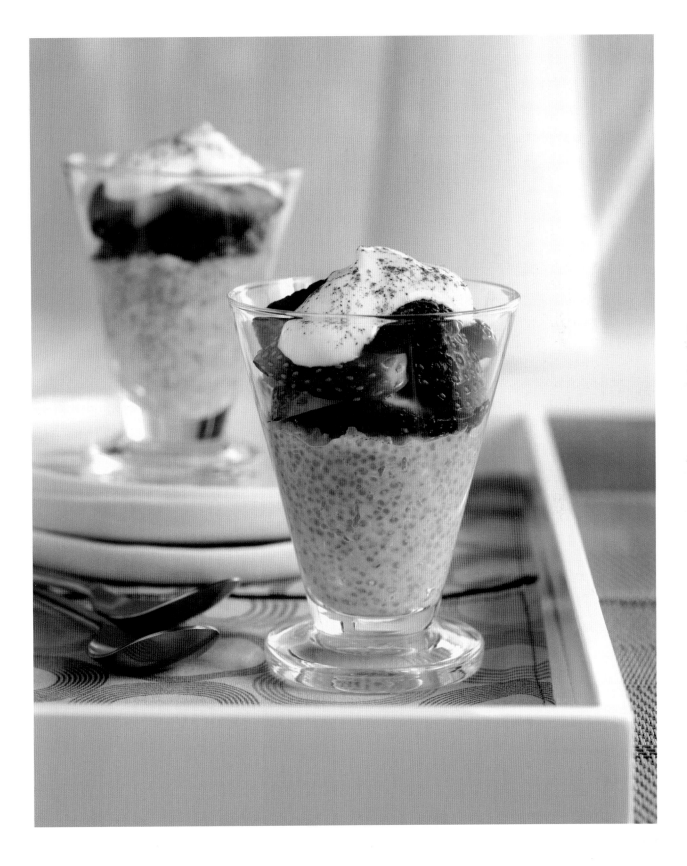

Watermelon Granita

vegan · **vegetarian** · dairy-free · **nut-free** · **gluten-free**

Makes 8 servings

5 cups cubed seeded watermelon

¼ cup agave nectar

1 tablespoon fresh lemon or lime juice

1. Place watermelon, agave and lemon juice in food processor; process until nearly smooth. Taste and add additional agave, if necessary.

2. Pour into 8-inch square baking dish. Cover and freeze about 5 hours or until firm.

3. Break watermelon mixture into chunks in baking dish. Freeze about 3 hours or until firm. To serve, stir and scrape granita with fork to create icy texture. Spoon into dessert dishes.

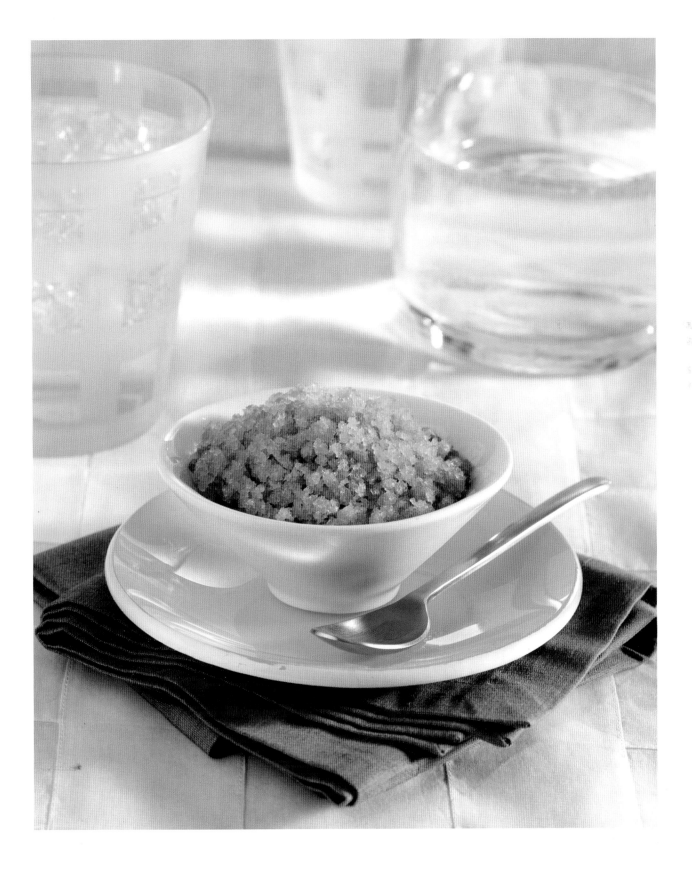

Spiced Vanilla Applesauce

vegan · **vegetarian** · dairy-free · **nut-free** · **gluten-free**

Makes 6 cups

5 **pounds (about 10 medium) apples (such as Fuji or Gala), peeled and cut into 1-inch pieces**

½ **cup water**

2 **teaspoons vanilla**

1 **teaspoon ground cinnamon**

¼ **teaspoon ground nutmeg**

¼ **teaspoon ground cloves**

1. Combine apples, water, vanilla, cinnamon, nutmeg and cloves in slow cooker; stir to blend. Cover; cook on HIGH 3 to 4 hours or until apples are very tender.

2. Turn off heat. Mash mixture with potato masher to smooth out any large lumps. Let cool completely before serving.

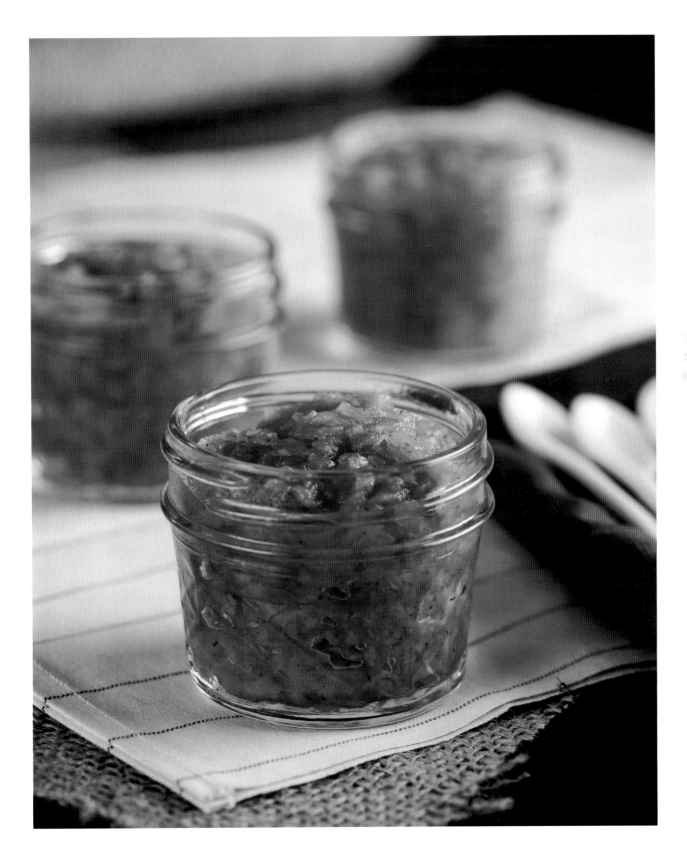

Speedy Pineapple-Lime Sorbet

vegan · **vegetarian** · dairy-free · **nut-free** · **gluten-free**

Makes 8 servings

1 ripe pineapple, cut into
   cubes (about 4 cups)

¼ cup fresh lime juice

1 teaspoon grated lime peel

1. Arrange pineapple in single layer on large baking sheet; freeze at least 1 hour or until very firm.*

2. Combine frozen pineapple, lime juice and lime peel in food processor or blender; process until smooth and fluffy. If mixture doesn't become smooth and fluffy, let stand 30 minutes to soften slightly; repeat processing. Serve immediately.

Pineapple can be frozen up to 1 month. Transfer frozen pineapple to resealable freezer food storage bags.

Note: This dessert is best if served immediately, but it can be made ahead, stored in the freezer and softened several minutes before serving.

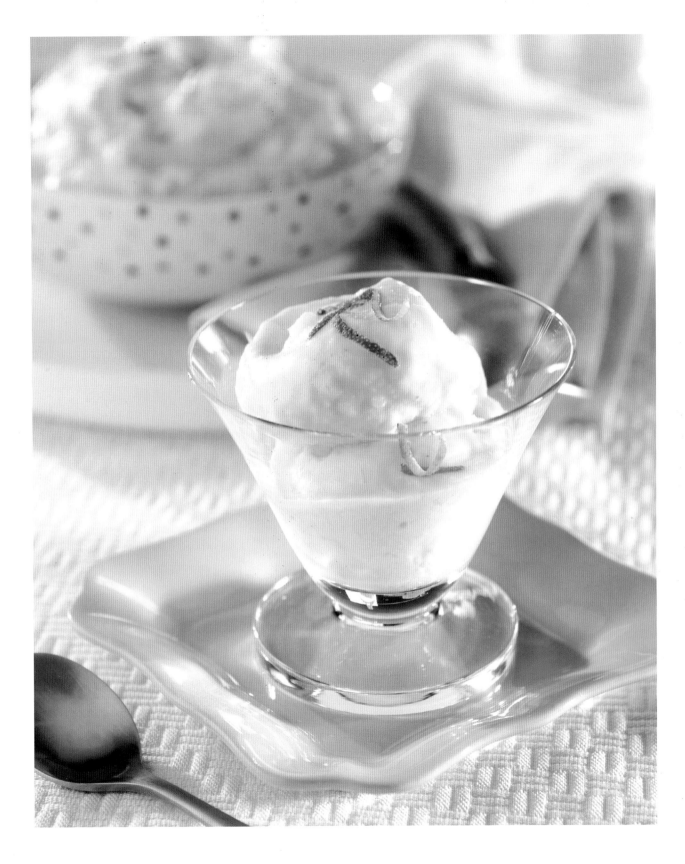

Index

Metric Conversion Chart

VOLUME MEASUREMENTS (dry)

1/8 teaspoon = 0.5 mL
1/4 teaspoon = 1 mL
1/2 teaspoon = 2 mL
3/4 teaspoon = 4 mL
1 teaspoon = 5 mL
1 tablespoon = 15 mL
2 tablespoons = 30 mL
1/4 cup = 60 mL
1/3 cup = 75 mL
1/2 cup = 125 mL
2/3 cup = 150 mL
3/4 cup = 175 mL
1 cup = 250 mL
2 cups = 1 pint = 500 mL
3 cups = 750 mL
4 cups = 1 quart = 1 L

VOLUME MEASUREMENTS (fluid)

1 fluid ounce (2 tablespoons) = 30 mL
4 fluid ounces (1/2 cup) = 125 mL
8 fluid ounces (1 cup) = 250 mL
12 fluid ounces (1 1/2 cups) = 375 mL
16 fluid ounces (2 cups) = 500 mL

WEIGHTS (mass)

1/2 ounce = 15 g
1 ounce = 30 g
3 ounces = 90 g
4 ounces = 120 g
8 ounces = 225 g
10 ounces = 285 g
12 ounces = 360 g
16 ounces = 1 pound = 450 g

DIMENSIONS

1/16 inch = 2 mm
1/8 inch = 3 mm
1/4 inch = 6 mm
1/2 inch = 1.5 cm
3/4 inch = 2 cm
1 inch = 2.5 cm

OVEN TEMPERATURES

250°F = 120°C
275°F = 140°C
300°F = 150°C
325°F = 160°C
350°F = 180°C
375°F = 190°C
400°F = 200°C
425°F = 220°C
450°F = 230°C

BAKING PAN SIZES

Utensil	Size in Inches/Quarts	Metric Volume	Size in Centimeters
Baking or Cake Pan (square or rectangular)	8×8×2	2 L	20×20×5
	9×9×2	2.5 L	23×23×5
	12×8×2	3 L	30×20×5
	13×9×2	3.5 L	33×23×5
Loaf Pan	8×4×3	1.5 L	20×10×7
	9×5×3	2 L	23×13×7
Round Layer Cake Pan	8×1½	1.2 L	20×4
	9×1½	1.5 L	23×4
Pie Plate	8×1¼	750 mL	20×3
	9×1¼	1 L	23×3
Baking Dish or Casserole	1 quart	1 L	—
	1½ quart	1.5 L	—
	2 quart	2 L	—